Insight Job

20 QUESTS FOR YOUR JOURNEY WITHIN

Insight Job
20 QUESTS FOR YOUR JOURNEY WITHIN

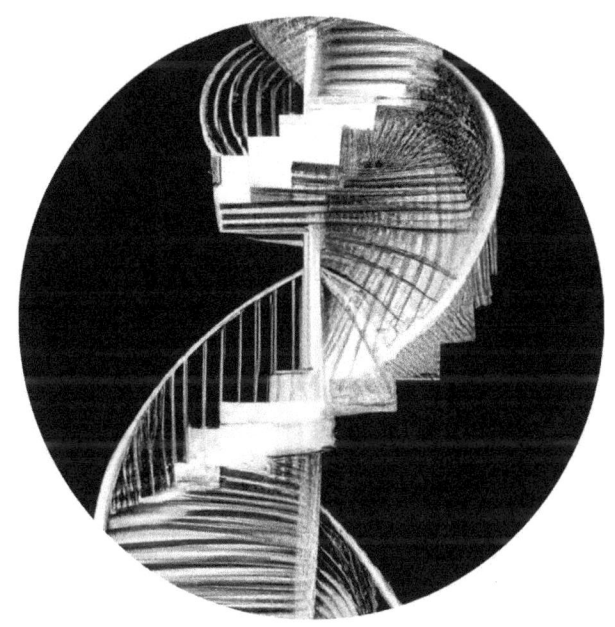

Aida I. Askry, Ph.D.

EDITED BY
Benjamin Schultz

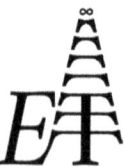

Evertree Publishing
www.evertreepublishing.com

Copyright © 2018, 2023

All rights reserved. No part of this book may be used or reproduced without written permission from the publisher except in the case of brief quotations.

Published 2023

ISBN 978-1-7321526-1-8

Printed in the United States of America

This journey is all yours.

Contents

Introduction		1
Chapter One		**11**
Quest 1A	Cultivate a Little Solitude	12
Quest 1B	Integumentary System	34
Quest 1C	Digestive System	40
Quest 1D	Muscular System	46
Quest 1E	Nervous System	54
Quest 1F	Immune System	59
Quest 1G	Skeletal System	68
Quest 1H	Endocrine System	74
Chapter Two		**85**
Quest 2A	What Do I Know?	88
Quest 2B	Cultivate a Little Mindfulness	92
Quest 2C	Conscious Mind	98
Quest 2D	Subconscious Mind	104
Quest 2E	Unconscious Mind	116
Chapter Three		**123**
Chapter Four		**133**
Quest 4A	Virtue of Authenticity	136
Quest 4B	Virtue of Understanding	148
Quest 4C	Virtue of Forgiveness	154
Quest 4D	Virtue of Allowance	162
Quest 4E	Virtue of Balance	170
Quest 4F	Virtue of Unity	179
Quest 4G	Virtue of Compassion	184

Introduction

HUMANITY is presently immersed in an extraordinary technological revolution. Connected instantaneously with friends and colleagues around the globe, we strive to cooperate as we watch the boundaries of our diverse native cultures rapidly fade away. Together, we are beginning to unfold the new possibilities and challenges provided by the integrated global culture forming before our collective eyes.

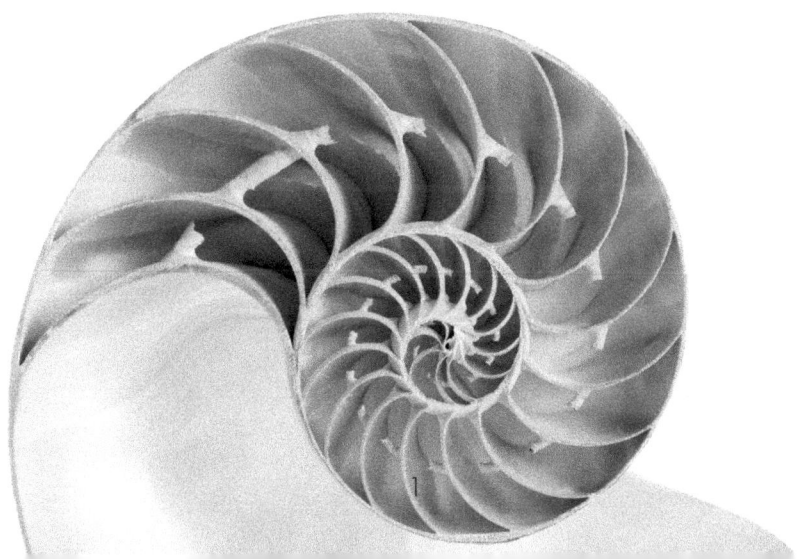

Insight Job

Through distributed scientific inquiry, we have called into question our deepest beliefs to re-establish our idea of the true nature of reality. We no longer receive guidance from ancestral traditions and community elders, relying instead on information compiled by highly specialized experts in every field of science and technology. Our species' technological evolution provides us with an expanded understanding of the human body's internal functions as well as closer glimpses of the surroundings outside our physical frame. From the smallest forms of existence (quarks, photons, atoms, and biological cells) to the largest mysteries of our convoluted universe (time and space, galaxies, energetic fields, and other unseen phenomena), we continually seek deeper knowledge for the sake of progress and to satisfy our natural curiosity. Using the data and innovation characteristic of this rapidly developing scientific era, we have not only changed the face of the Earth but also our understanding of ourselves: present, future, and perhaps past, too.

By contrast, our ancestors' deep wisdom which guided them to create monumental wonders of construction and inscription that still captivate us today arose primarily from their ancient cultural knowledge and profound philosophical self-understanding. Many of these traditions teach that the human form contains three major components: "body," "mind," and "spirit" (which different viewpoints refer to as soul, higher self, essence, life force, pure consciousness, Chi, and Prana). Some advise limiting our physical needs and desires for the sake of the non-physical. Others teach techniques to develop our mental and physical body in preparation for the experience of higher states of being. Teachings from around the world and throughout time contain many similarities, but the specific methods and recommendations employed by each tradition vary widely. These inconsistencies, combined with the conflicting messages presented in today's information-dense world, can make it difficult for the individual to define a personal path of growth.

Introduction

The teachings available to us alive today will often separate body, mind, or spirit—seeking the maximum potential in only one plane of existence. Religions look to messages of the past, providing varying explanations of our history and presenting a story of personal responsibility for our spiritual growth. Science looks to the future, hoping to reveal the mysteries of our world and put them to work for our physical benefit. Societal pressures and keen marketing imagery vie to impregnate our subconscious mind with uninvited desires. Meanwhile, each of us engages daily in an all-encompassing life experience that never ceases to challenge every dimension of our being. While scientific objectivism may persuade many to dismiss mental, emotional, or "spiritual" (multidimensional) discipline and clarity as unverifiable, subjective—and, hence, irrelevant— traits, even cursory introspection reveals the health of these dimensions of our existence to be both fundamental and essential to the state of our well-being and the quality of our decision-making.

Despite their perceived differences, the fields of science, philosophy, and even spirituality have always shared a common desire to comprehend the true nature of this reality with which we interact every day. Science has demonstrated that, with increased comprehension of our physical reality, we can change the way we experience this world. Similarly, philosophical comprehension and understanding expands the domain of possibilities for the body, mind, and spirit. As the true nature of reality is intertwined with the wisdom of philosophy and the intelligence of science, our complete understanding cannot ignore the philosophical and spiritual wisdom of the past, nor the scientific intelligence of the future. Thus, the separation of philosophy and science is a superstition. It is the harmony of both viewpoints that is essential for mankind's development. Although it appears that our possibilities are limited by the conditions of time and space, our rightful focus on the present moment will expose our true potential.

Insight Job

As Baba Ram Dass would say,

"Be here now."[1]

We have only one way to participate in the present moment: re-present all three dimensions of the whole human being as one. These three dimensions create one's true self without any false perception of separation. Transpersonal psychologist Dr. James Strohl writes,

> *Human beings are considered multidimensional entities because, while living our lives on Earth, we simultaneously maintain physical and nonphysical presences or aspects of ourselves in many other realities. All of these presences, including our current human one, are conscious components or aspects of a larger, super-conscious multidimensional self which is sometimes called inner being or soul. Even though these aspects of our multidimensional inner being are manifesting innumerous different physical and nonphysical worlds, they can communicate and influence each other while also retaining a deep and abiding connection to inner being.*[2]

As we begin to comprehend the relation between spirit, mind, and body, we inevitably feel a need to seek a path of practice for growth and development in all three aspects. To participate in the present moment with all dimensions of your self, you must find a path or make your own. *Insight Job* is designed to support you, regardless of your belief system, through a deeper exploration of the true nature of your own consciousness, mind, and body, so you may reveal your own pragmatic path of experience and understanding to guide you through your life journey.

Introduction

How to Use This Book

Insight Job combines mental, physical, and metaphysical practices collected from masters and experts who unveiled their multidimensional true selves to be wholeheartedly present, balancing their human lives as a whole. The following chapters explore the principles behind these practices while offering twenty inner quests to assist you in your journey toward balance of spirit, mind, and body as a multidimensional being.

The main print of this book appears succinct because you create density of information internally with your own practice of awareness. Self-transformation can come only from within your unique self. It's an inside job. As we will discuss in Chapter Two, conscious knowing alone cannot change subconscious patterns. Instead, a deeper understanding is essential—insight that can grow only from experience and repeated practice.

We all have different life situations, histories, and goals that we bring to the present moment. Each chapter of this book provides practices to be adapted to your own life. The written explanation of each practice serves as a foundation. Beyond that, you have the liberty to define your practice to suit your needs. If uncertain about the specific formulation of your practice, it is always helpful to look within. Ask your heart how to build your practice based on what you feel you truly need. Sometimes the practice you need is the opposite of the practice you naturally want. And because any rigid pattern breaks under stress, do not treat your practices as a chore you must complete or an inflexible framework that cannot evolve or change. Approach your practice with childlike wonder and ingenuity. With a true desire for understanding, you will learn as quickly and deeply as a child. Forge ahead in your present moment, as the process of self-understanding—understanding the deeper reality of your existence in this universe—will provide you with a greater sense of purpose, adventure, and joy of experience than can be found in any man-made distraction.

Your life experience is complex and ever-changing. For this reason, your journey will certainly require employing resources beyond this book, especially during Chapter One which explores physical concepts well-documented by our scientific society. We are fortunate to live in a time of connection. We can connect locally with skilled practitioners for services or support, and we can connect instantly to detailed, up-to-date information online. Both resources should be utilized as needed to support your journey. It is not possible to present the tasks in this book as check-the-box exercises that provide you all the answers. This is simply because your answers will be unique to your own experience and situation. You can build and support your journey using any knowledge available to you. Connect with your world. Everything comes easily with the right connections.

Dedicated application of the practices presented here leads toward a fully integrated human experience. As such, the practices themselves are integrated and co-related. You're asked to progress through this book sequentially, practicing under each chapter's given instructions and discipline, moving forward only when you honestly feel suitably proficient and ready to continue to the next chapter. Being honest with yourself is the first key to decoding the embedded patterns and beliefs that keep you from evolving beyond your current state of understanding. Proceed at your own pace. This is a process of natural growth. Savor all your practices as you explore your own story, chapter by chapter.

Introduction

The first two chapters of this book contain physical and mental practices that bring your awareness more firmly into your body and mind. At the end of each quest, the book provides space to record your first practice and shape your next. You may want to repeat some of the quests a number of times before moving on. In this case, you can dedicate a notebook of your choosing as your Quest Log to record your continued experiences. Because your Quest Log holds personal observations of your physical and mental development over time, is the most important part of this book.

Insight Job is not the type of book you can put down for months with hopes to return later, nor the type of book that can be loaned to a friend. This is your book and your inside story. It is asking to be read and written, without judgment or fear of being right or wrong. Your story will return to you all the attention and love you invest in it. You're not reading to distract yourself from past or future events. You are writing your own journey through the present moment.

Planting the Seed

Before you begin this journey, set your intention for your practice. Taking inspiration from the universe right outside the door, imagine yourself as a gardener planting a tree of inner health and balance. Your intention to grow a beautiful life experience plants the seed of your "Tree of Life." Thoughts and actions can nourish your tree or promote weeds. Trust that your supportive thoughts and mindful actions will nurture your seed into a sapling that you will care for and enjoy as it grows into a distinctively beautiful tree.

Looking deeper, we see that the tree is grounded in your belief system existing as roots that absorb sustenance from the external world. Growing upwards, your spirit forms a sturdy or flexible trunk upon which your physical and mental health grow as bark and limbs. Branches, provided with strength and nutrition from the limbs, represent family, social life, hobbies, and your career. Many people dedicate substantial time and energy to fixing or perfecting the form of the branches while forgetting to take care of the trunk and the roots. It's no wonder their branches sometimes dry out. Fortunately, when you focus on nourishing the roots and your spirit first, the branches will naturally flourish.

Chapter One focuses on our physical health to plant the seed of our practice in a positive environment. Once the sapling has taken root, we will see it flourish through Chapters Two, Three, and Four where we explore the workings of the inner self. Do not be discouraged if your sapling does not flower immediately, or even if it has trouble taking root. Patience and persistent care, especially during times of harsh climate, will inevitably allow your tree to grow at its natural pace, eventually presenting fruits of skill and wisdom beyond all expectation.

Introduction

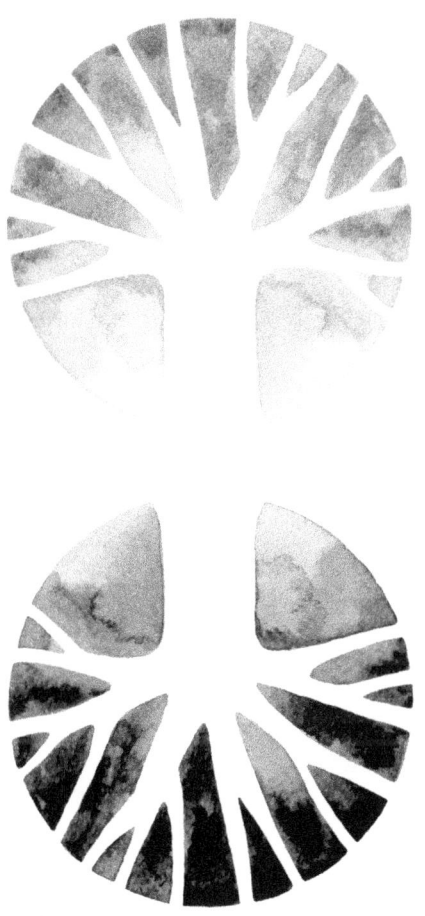

End of Introduction

Chapter One
HUMAN BODY

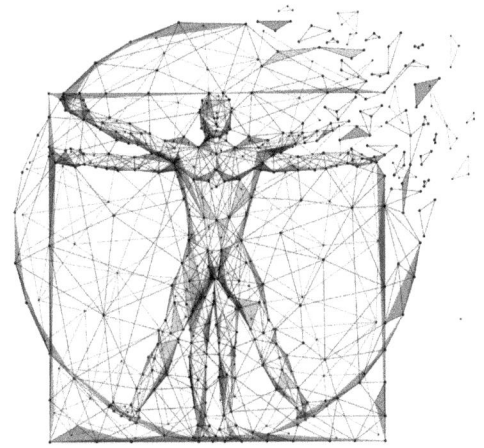

THE JOURNEY through your *Insight Job* is propelled by awareness, navigated by understanding, and safeguarded by compassion and acceptance. Through this adventure you can expect to cultivate wisdom by necessity as your awareness of your self, your world, and your universe grows stronger.

Leave uncertainty behind and dive within, without fear, to a quest focused on cultivating awareness of the physical body that serves to carry out your worldly actions. In the following practice, you will explore and document the soil in which you are planting your Tree of Life.

QUEST 1A
CULTIVATE A LITTLE SOLITUDE

Observation

Start by finding yourself a comfortable place to sit and relax. Once seated, simply observe your current physical state without judgment or manipulation. Delicately focus your awareness on the following sensations:

- breathing pattern (quality of the breath: speed, depth, ease, ...)
- heart rate
- body temperature
- blood pressure
- posture
- feelings of heaviness or lightness
- digestive and abdominal sensations
- joint, skin, and muscular comfort or discomfort
- your overall state of physical health

In this state of awareness, your goal is to observe as much as possible, gently gathering information about the current state of being of your physical self.

Afterward, record your findings in your Quest Log. Keeping a record of this and all other practices in this book will prove invaluable as you unfold your true self. As you progress, your experience will feel so natural that it may be difficult to internalize a perspective of your growth without reviewing a firsthand account of your past experience.

Duration and Frequency

This quest could take 5 to 10 minutes or longer. No need to set a timer. Your task is simply to observe. As with any observation of a complex system, the longer you watch, the more information you will collect.

Use this opportunity to dedicate a small but expandable window of time in your daily routine that will create space for the practices in this book. Most practices in this book require no longer than 20 minutes; however, you're likely to naturally expand this window as your time with yourself becomes increasingly valuable and enjoyable.

For Quest 1A, it is up to you to define the frequency. Gather as much knowledge as you desire until you are comfortable moving on to the next quest. You may continue this practice alongside other quests in this book or return to it at any time to witness your present experience of self-awareness. You may be pleasantly surprised when new sensations reveal themselves as your awareness expands and your Tree of Life grows. Comfortable or not, remember to always greet these valuable new messages from your body with the respect they deserve.

Insight Job

QUEST LOG 1A
DAY ONE

Date:

Breathing pattern:

Heart rate & blood pressure:

Body temperature:

Heaviness or lightness:

Digestive & abdominal sensations:

Posture:

Chapter One: Human Body

QUEST LOG 1A

Joint/skin/muscle sensations:

Overall state of physical health & other observations:

While most of us are busy catching up with our professional life or our multitude of other responsibilities and commitments, we fail to notice or acknowledge the gradual changes of our personal health, physical body, or even our state of mind. Being conditioned to point our attention externally, many of us have completely forgotten how it feels to relax, enjoy a dull moment, or eat and sleep well. Even those of us in relatively affluent situations have often forgotten how to be present to enjoy the beautiful experience we have created so diligently. While using our intellect and advanced technology to create countless wonders from our planet's physical resources, we often fail to employ the same aptitude to discovering and exploring our true nature of being, seeing our physical, mental, and emotional health as it exists within this ecosystem.

Physical and mental health have far-reaching effects on the overall experience of life. Ancient cultures, defined the body as the vehicle for the mind and soul. Each philosophy developed or adopted its own set of rules, including dietary guidelines and physical activities (sometimes in the form of prayers), to maintain this vehicle—or "temple"—that is hosting the pure consciousness.

The quests you will explore over the following weeks, intended to be practiced as consciously and persistently as possible, serve to build your temple's foundation. They bring into conscious awareness the current state of balance in each system of your physical body. Expect to get more in touch with your posture, breath quality, sleep cycle, eating patterns, stress levels, and environmental health (including light, temperature, air quality, sounds, and exposure to nature). Only after spending some time understanding and cultivating our soil can we confidently watch our tree grow. Do not be overly concerned if you find your foundation in need of care. Increased awareness naturally stimulates the gradual lifestyle changes necessary to bring the physical body into balance.

Chapter One: Human Body

Human Body Systems

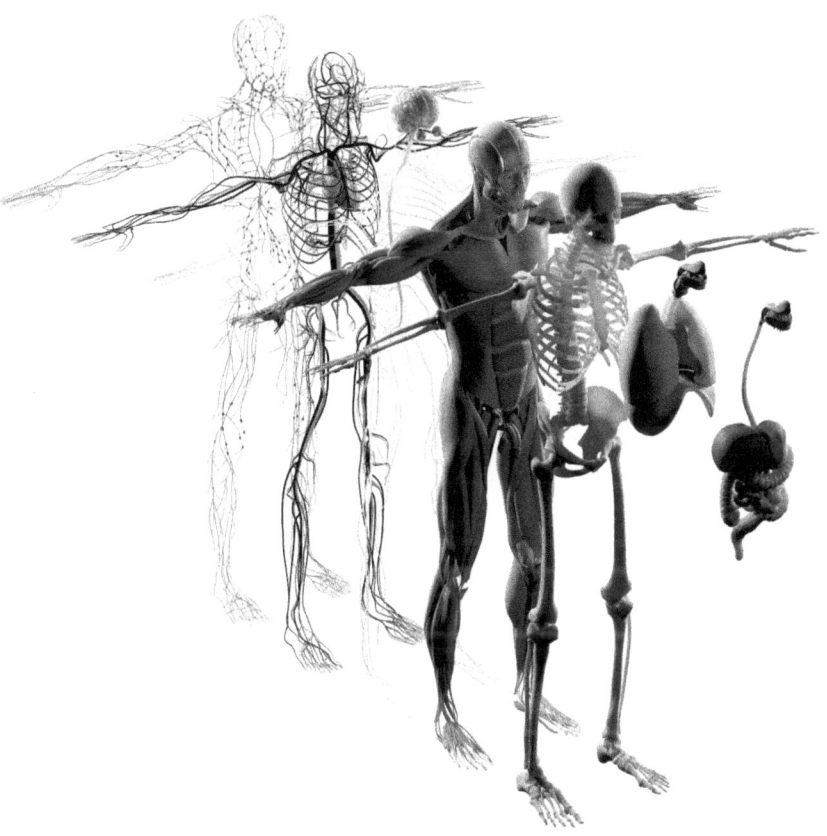

It may already be clear that each component of your self is comprised of interdependent subsystems, each of which requiring at least some attention. The physical human body is the most tangible and well-understood example. Most of us are very aware of what overt dysfunction or dis-ease in certain body systems can feel like: skin rashes, digestive distress, respiratory cough or congestion, and muscle soreness or tension.

However, imbalance in the less-palpable—but equally important—body systems can be more difficult to distinguish. How many of us can identify symptoms of dysfunction in the endocrine system? What state has your nervous system been living in lately? Your physical body depends on the overall state of health of your lifestyle and all body systems to operate well as a whole. Healthcare viewed through this lens is commonly known as the field of integrative medicine.

To make the deeper practices of self-discovery that you will explore in later chapters as comfortable as possible, we must first form a decent balance in all underlying physical systems. Of course, each system can be—and has been—studied on its own for an entire lifetime; however, even a general awareness of each main system, its needs, and its current state of health can be instrumental in creating balance.

The figures that follow give an overview of the body's major systems, including a description of each system's functions. As you review them, do your best to consciously feel the sensations associated with each system in your own body. By directing your focus inward, you allow your body to create neural connections that can eventually provide you with very precise information about each system's state of health. The value of this internal information is immeasurable. If you can act on subtle cues from within, then you gain the power to prevent minor dysfunction from escalating to painful disease.

Chapter One: Human Body

Integumentary System

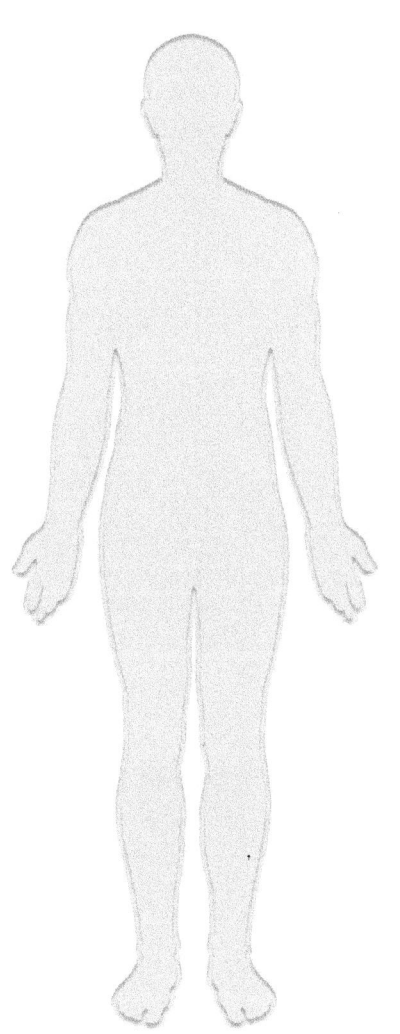

- Comprised of the skin: the largest organ in the body (2 square meters or 22 square feet of surface area)

- Provides sensation

- Serves as a barrier against infection, ultraviolet damage, and mechanical abrasion

- Contains sweat glands (and occasionally goosebumps) which regulate body temperature

- Synthesizes Vitamin D for use in other systems

Insight Job

Skeletal System

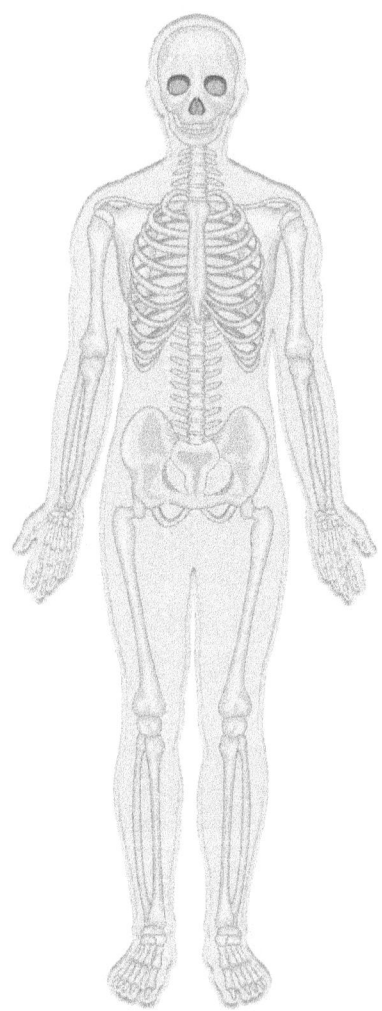

- Comprised of 206 bones and a variety of unique joints

- Allows the body to rise above the ground and stand upright

- Serves as the mineralized internal framework of the body

- Protects vital organs

- Provides the scaffolding for movement force generated by the muscular system

- Stores calcium, accumulating or releasing ions (as directed by the endocrine system) to balance blood plasma calcium concentration

- Produces red and white blood cells

Chapter One: Human Body

Muscular System

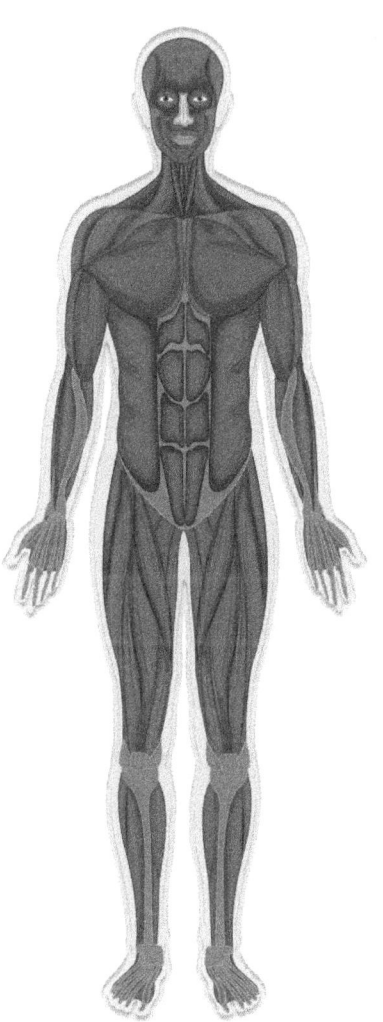

- Comprised of muscles that generate movement as well as connective tissues such as tendons and ligaments (the combined system of bones, muscles, and connective tissue is known as the "musculoskeletal system")

- Assists circulation

- Aids digestion

- Generates facial expressions

- Maintains posture

- Contracts to protect the body against perceived threats or discomfort

Cardiovascular System

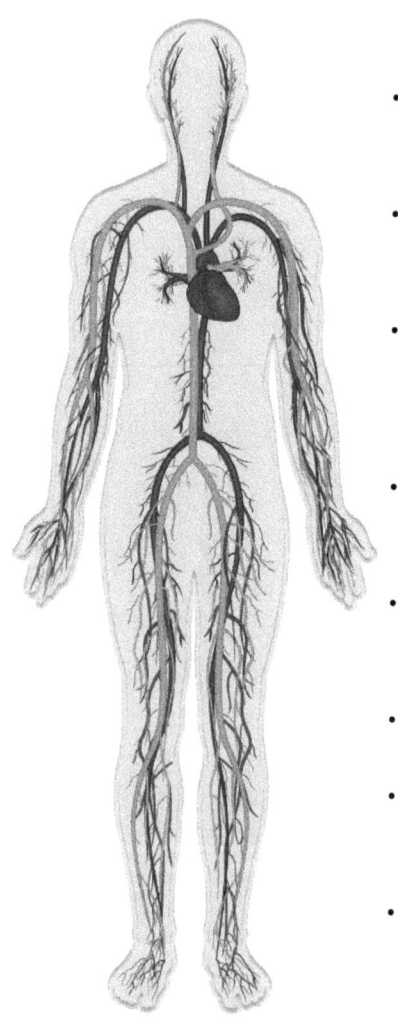

- Comprised of the heart and blood vessels

- Transports sustenance to every cell of the body

- Absorbs and transports oxygen and nutrients throughout the body

- Absorbs and transports cell waste

- Contains antibodies and immune cells

- Maintains pH of the body

- Contributes to temperature regulation

- Carries chemical messengers (hormones) produced by the endocrine system

Chapter One: Human Body

Lymphatic System

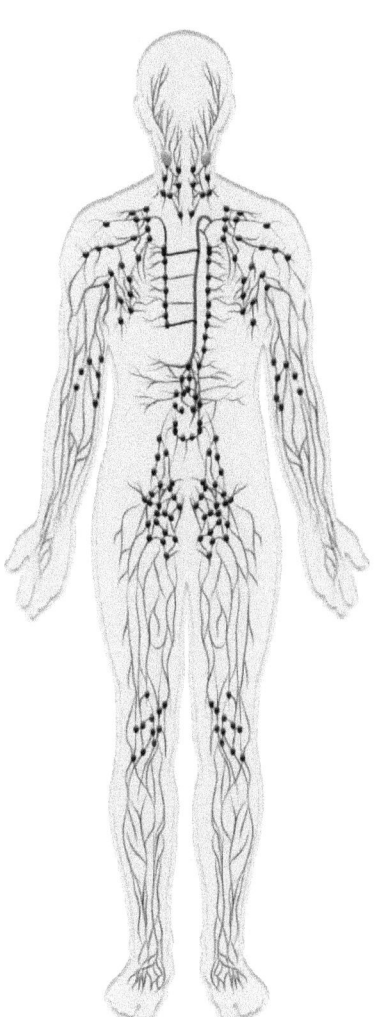

- Comprised of interstitial fluid, an open-ended network of tubular vessels, lymph nodes, and organs including the tonsils, spleen, and thymus

- Circulates interstitial fluid, which consists of water, ions, and solutes (small particles) that constantly diffuse from the blood through the walls of capillaries, unidirectionally toward the heart

- Lymph nodes trap and destroy pathogens, damaged cells, and cancerous cells

- Houses lymphocytes, a group of white blood cells that support immunity

- Maintains fluid balance between tissues and blood vessels

Nervous System

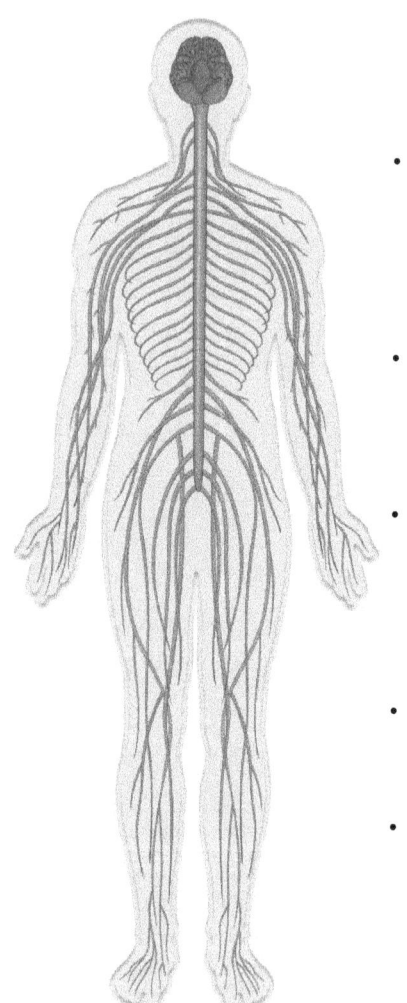

- Comprised of the brain and spinal cord, nerves and neurons, along with the primary sense organs

- Maintains internal order, coordinating actions of the muscles and organs

- Receives and interprets sensory input, triggers reactions, and provides protection from danger

- Supports learning and understanding

- Shifts the body between "fight or flight" and "rest and repair" modes

Respiratory System

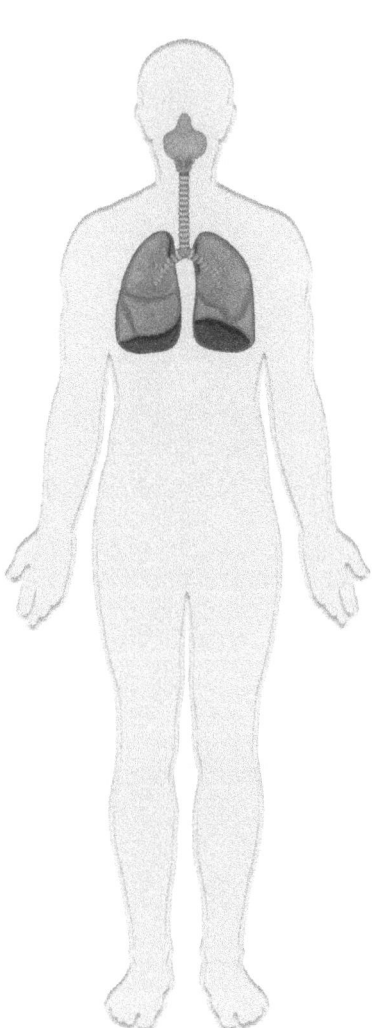

- Comprised of the lungs, tubes to carry air to and from the lungs, and the muscles of respiration (the diaphragm and intercostal muscles in the ribs)

- Exchanges gases: brings oxygen into the body and releases carbon dioxide

- Supports sound generation and speech

- Protects body from invasion by airborne pathogens

Digestive System

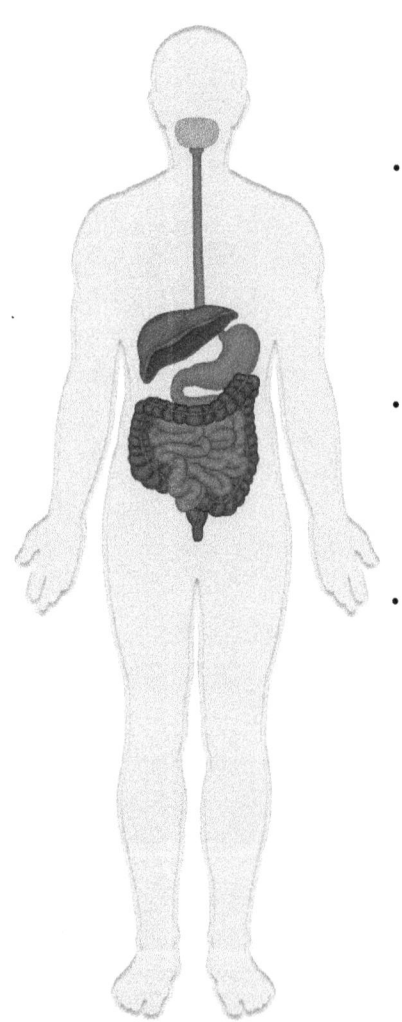

- Comprised of the mouth, esophagus, stomach, liver, gallbladder, pancreas, small intestine, and large intestine (colon and rectum)

- Responsible for breaking down food into the building blocks of the body, then absorbing and assimilating these nutrients

- Houses the gut flora: multitudes of beneficial microorganisms (the "microbiome") responsible for synthesizing some vitamins and supporting immune function

Chapter One: Human Body

Urinary System

- Comprised of the kidneys and bladder

- Cleans dissolved waste products from the blood

- Excretes liquid waste

- Regulates electrolytes, fluid, and pH balance

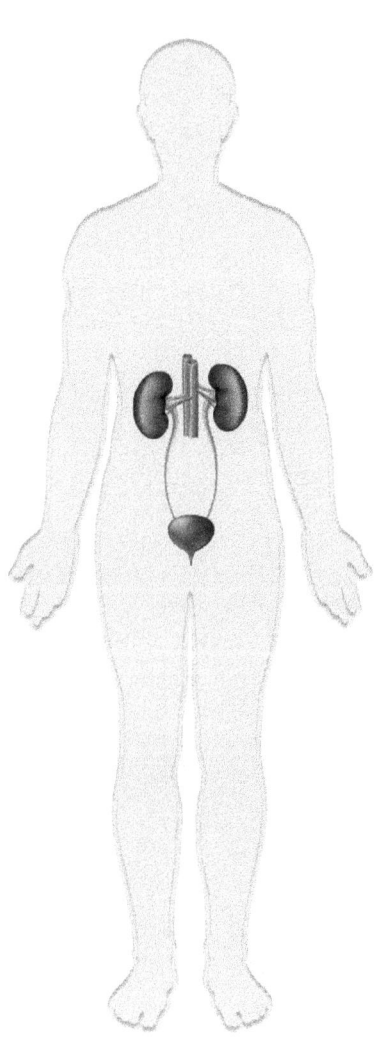

Endocrine System

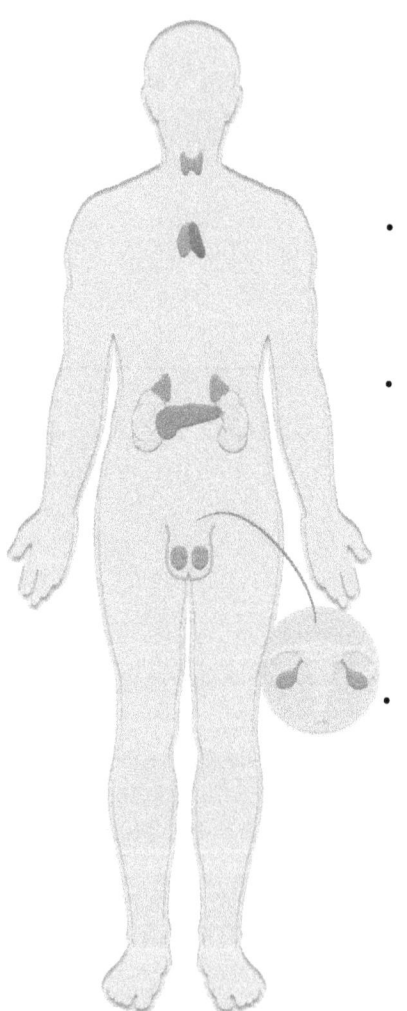

- Comprised of a series of glands that secrete hormones into the circulatory system

- Involved in every process of the body, hormones act as chemical messengers that regulate growth, metabolic activity, nutrient utilization, mineral retention, sleep cycles, and many other bodily functions

- Involved in development and maturation of the adaptive immune system

Chapter One: Human Body

Reproductive System

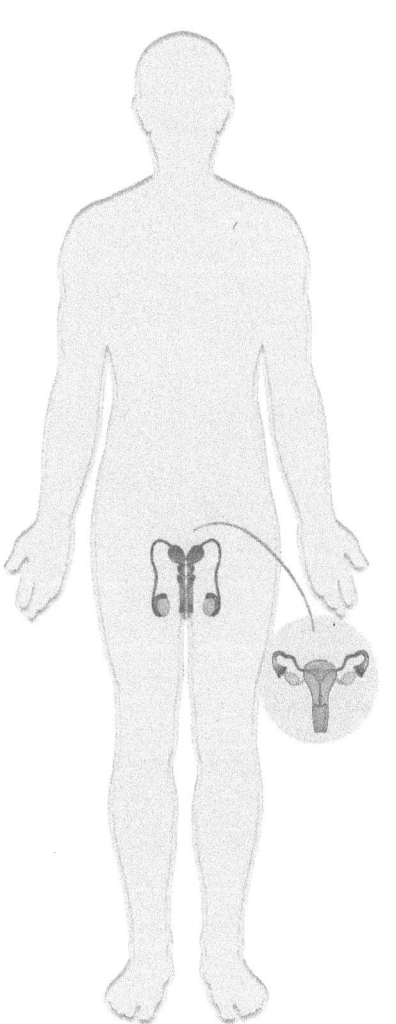

- Comprised of the ovaries, uterus, and mammary glands in women and the penis, prostate, and testes in men

- Allows the production of offspring

Immune System

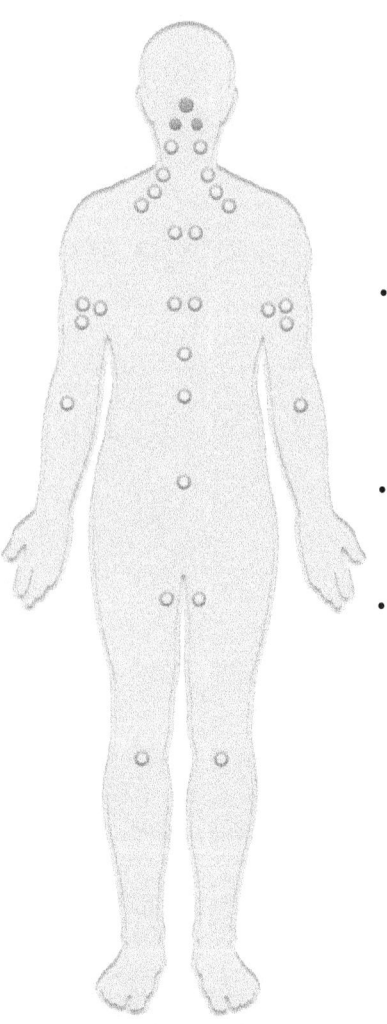

- Comprised of the portions of other systems that filter, identify, disable, or remove pathogens

- Depends strongly on the lymphatic system

- Relies on the proper function of all other systems

Chapter One: Human Body

Human Body System Practices

By becoming more aware of your physical form and the systems therein, you are allowing the energy of your thoughts, actions, and your body's internal healing mechanisms to flow towards those areas that need attention. The following practices will guide and remind you to take simple, harmonious steps to take care of your physical body.

Although there is no magic pill to balance the body overnight, each evening you can review that day's actions to make sure you are gradually drawing closer to the goal(s) you set for yourself with your intention. With each day's practice, you reinforce a healing habit that becomes increasingly effortless as it is ingrained in your natural tendencies. The following practices may take weeks or months; but you're encouraged to take your time and focus on each practice until you begin to experience noticeable improvements. You can take full credit for these changes because your awareness and actions were responsible for them. You should notice simple improvements almost immediately, as the body often requires only a little push to be brought back into a balanced, healing state. Healthy body systems provide better support for healing each other. All the quests in this book reinforce each other through this advantageous relationship. As each system comes into balance, it requires fewer resources to maintain. Spare energy is naturally utilized by the body to repair other systems until balance is restored to the point that more energy can be directed to higher faculties of conscious, creative action.

Be mindful that the objective of these practices is to enhance self-awareness. Do not obsess over the body or physical results. Find the balance between awareness and hyperawareness. Take your time and avoid wasting energy comparing yourself to others or looking for shortcuts. This is neither a race nor a competition.

Practice each quest for at least one week and up to three weeks. Explore what works best for you. Let yourself have fun with your practice as you experience contentment in awareness and delight in improvement.

Chapter One: Human Body

Week One: Integumentary System

Starting with the system that is responsible for the largest organ in the human body, becoming mindful of your skin allows you to find simple and effective improvements that are noticeable, touchable and rewarding.

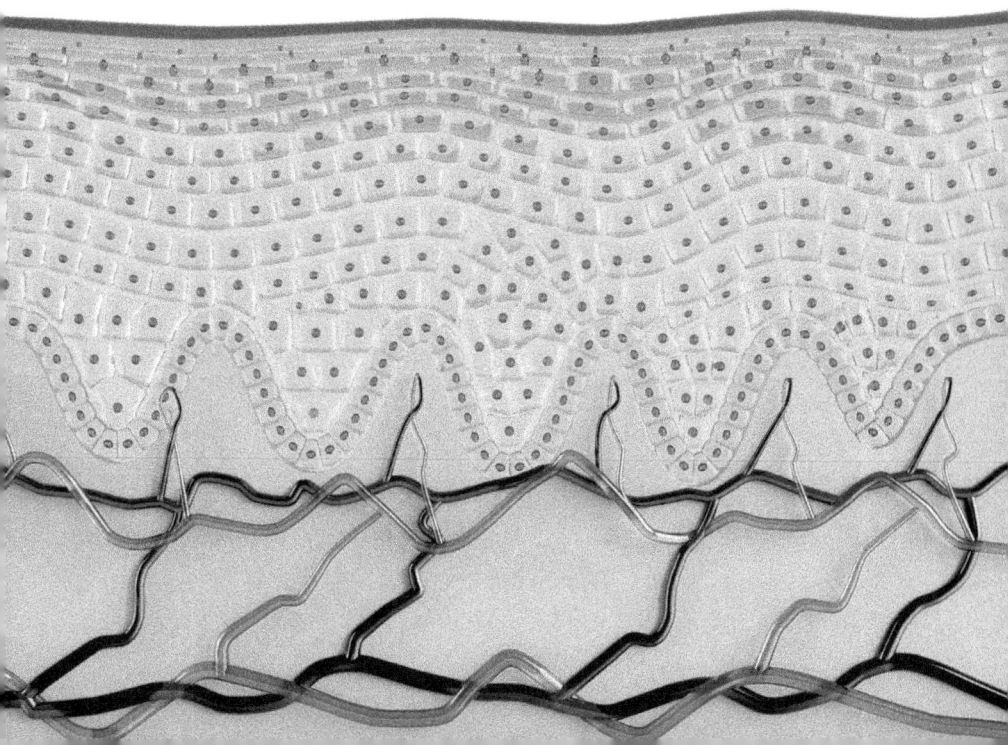

QUEST 1B
INTEGUMENTARY SYSTEM

In this quest and throughout the rest of this chapter, you will better understand how the physical systems of the human body are formed in co-operation with each other and are all interdependent. Dermatologists and other professional skincare specialists would be first ones to tell you that skin care starts from your gut. Later we will focus on how you can support your digestive system, but for this first week, start by observing your skin from head to toe. Ask yourself: *How could I protect myself from damage and enhance the quality of my skin?* In this week's daily routine, spend a bit more effort mindfully observing and caring for your skin.

Observation

Begin by simply taking a closer look at your skin, hair, and nails. Touch your skin from the outside and feel it from within, taking note of its appearance, texture, and sensation.

Action

After allowing your skin to communicate with you through sight and touch, set your own short-term goal for your skin. As with all goals in the following practices, our skin care goal needs to be "SMART," conforming to the following criteria: Specific, Measurable, Attainable, Relevant and Timely.

Protection:

After setting a goal, begin your practice of skin protection. You can use methods or products with which you are already familiar or connect with a friend or the Internet to seek recommendations. Choose one or two natural methods that can help you protect your skin from damage by natural sources (such as the sun), or by unnatural sources (such as chemicals and pollutants).

Nourishment and Enhancement:

If you are already maintaining protection methods, then it's time to enhance your practice and nurture your skin with natural oils or supplements. You may begin applying this immediately or complete the first week of observation and protection practice first.

Duration and Frequency

Focus on skin protection as often as possible during your daily activities. Use your chosen nourishment and enhancement methods at least daily or as required.

Practice for one to three weeks. Observation and protection may be practiced for some time before nourishment and enhancement begin. Enjoy the improvements day by day.

Insight Job

QUEST LOG 1B
DAY ONE

Date:

Observations: (skin texture, pigmentation, dryness/oiliness, comfort, ...)

Skincare goal: (specific, measurable, attainable, relevant, timely)

Today's protection methods:

Today's nourishment & enhancement methods:

Concepts deserving further study or practice:

Chapter One: Human Body

QUEST LOG 1B
DAY TWO

Date:

Observations & improvements:

Status of goal:

Today's protection methods:

Today's nourishment & enhancement methods:

Concepts deserving further study or practice:

Week Two: Digestive System

The digestive system plays an important role in our health. It is through this system that we break down the food we have consciously chosen to eat into its constituent nutrients that inform our cells with the building blocks required for repair and growth.

One common misunderstanding is to confuse digestive improvement with metabolic enhancement. Digestive organs, from the mouth to the colon, are responsible for properly breaking down food, eliminating food waste, and sending nutrients into the body in the forms of proteins, carbohydrates, and lipids. Metabolism, regulated by the endocrine and nervous systems, is cells' ability to convert these nutrients, existing in the form of potential chemical energy, into kinetic energy that can move the body, grow cells, and repair tissues inside the body.

Remember, "empty" calories (foods that provide energy or flavor, but contain limited nutritional building blocks) do not provide the restorative nutrients the body uses for cell construction and maintenance. Missing or imbalanced building blocks, especially combined with environmental stressors, can lead your body to crave even more food. Unless the body's requests are satisfied with legitimate nutrition, enjoyed mindfully, the extra energy content in empty calories may be stored in fat cells, while other systems of the body work overtime to process artificial ingredients, preservatives, sweeteners, and other extraneous compounds.

Conscious eating is a popular form of mindfulness, because most of us have the good fortune to be able to choose what we eat every single day. We can be mindful not only of the flavor of food, but also character of its nutrients. Once we understand what foods will nourish the body and acknowledge the substances that may harm our being, a desire to

Chapter One: Human Body

control the quality of our nutrition grows naturally. Through this wisdom, we can appreciate the value of choosing foods that are generative and healing for the body as well as intricately pleasurable to consume. It is then intuitive to avoid ingesting foods and substances that provide only convenience or superficial pleasure then create uncomfortable states of body or mind thereafter. This isn't forcing a diet or counting calories, but rather considering nutrients and caring for yourself. Let your intelligence and desire for health guide your actions.

While nutritional advice can be inconsistent and often changes over time, you can always perceptively observe your own body's reaction to simple changes in food intake. This week, you will take the simple step of adding or taking away food groups or substances from your daily eating plan. Let's be SMART again. Set a goal of repaying your cells for their tireless efforts by giving them what they need.

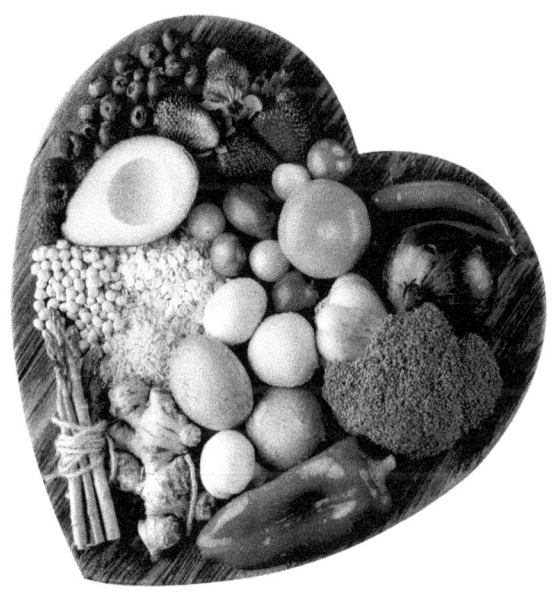

QUEST 1C
DIGESTIVE SYSTEM

Observation

Take some time to observe your daily eating patterns. Being aware of the true needs of your body in terms of digestion and metabolism, what could you mindfully add to or take away from your diet for a period of time?

Action

Write your SMART goal and make the honest decision to achieve it. This could be as simple as drinking four extra cups of water per day or eliminating a major food category (consider sugar, alcohol, gluten, caffeine, or animal products) for a period of time. The goal of this practice is to support your digestive system by becoming mindful of your eating habits and perhaps making lifestyle changes, as opposed to imposing a temporary diet. You may not lose weight as a result of this practice, but you will certainly gain more insight into your body's reaction to what you choose to ingest.

You could also use this quest as an opportunity to prepare more food at home, focusing on consuming whole foods and natural herbs or spices, while avoiding processed food and additives. Not only does this guarantee you exact knowledge and control of the ingredients in your food, it may also give you an opportunity to spend more quality time with family, friends, or loved ones. Your state of mind, along with the environment in which your meal is consumed, can influence your body's response as much as the food itself.

Duration and Frequency

Try to be mindful of every piece of food you consume. Even if you continue eating some less nutritious foods, acknowledging them as such can naturally affect your eating decisions over time.

Write your first Quest Log after spending adequate time observing and setting a goal, then continue with your next log at the end of each day to track your progress.

Set a goal you can achieve, choosing a change you can maintain. Modify your eating patterns for at least seven days, but preferably twenty-one days. This gives your body time to readjust to new patterns and, if applicable, purge the chemical effects of addictive substances. After this time, consider whether you want to continue, modify, or improve your practice.

Insight Job

QUEST LOG 1C
DAY ONE

Date:

Observations about current eating patterns:
(quality, quantity, excessive or underutilized food groups)

Digestive system goal:
(What to remove? What to add? What to focus on? SMART)

Concepts deserving further study or practice:

Chapter One: Human Body

QUEST LOG 1C
DAY TWO

Date:

Today's food intake: (list of foods or food groups)

Digestive system reaction and potential causes:
(What factors may have contributed? Quality or quantity of food? Stress?)

Status of goal:

Focus areas for tomorrow's practice:

Concepts deserving further study or practice:

Insight Job

Week Three: Muscular System

One of the most commonly known systems of the human body is the muscular system. Unfortunately, that also means it is one of the systems most often unintentionally abused or misused. Even today, many healthcare professionals and trainers do not fully comprehend the natural functionality and responsibilities of the muscular system, but rather focus on visibly re-shaping the muscles and isolating muscle groups independently. Your muscular system is not only responsible for physical appearance, movement, and mobility, but also plays a significant role in digestion and the circulation of blood (and other fluids) into different parts of the body. Supportive of posture, including emotionally and physically protective postures that can become habitual, your muscular health can also reveal much about the health of your emotional body. This means you can work with your muscular system to release emotional stress and tension or work with your emotional body to relieve chronic physical pain.

The musculoskeletal system covers the entire body, head to toe, with multiple layers of musculature enfolded within. The deepest and most powerful layers are often responsible for integrating movement of the appendages (arms, legs, neck and head) with the stability of the core (hips, shoulders, and torso). When properly activated and balanced, all muscles work together to create efficient and coherent motion that does not easily cause fatigue or joint damage. For most people living in today's world, the deepest layers of the muscular system are locked in perpetual tension (exacerbated by excessive sitting and deep emotional holding), leaving only the superficial muscles to perform body movements. This leads us to chronic muscle and joint pain, feelings of exhaustion and weakness, and difficulty expressing ourselves physically and emotionally. Fortunately, strength, stamina, and a feeling of expansiveness can be gained by simply unraveling this deep-seated muscular tension. Methods for releasing this

Chapter One: Human Body

tension will become more apparent as you connect with your whole being on every level. The reward of lightness and freedom within your body is well worth the effort of exploration.

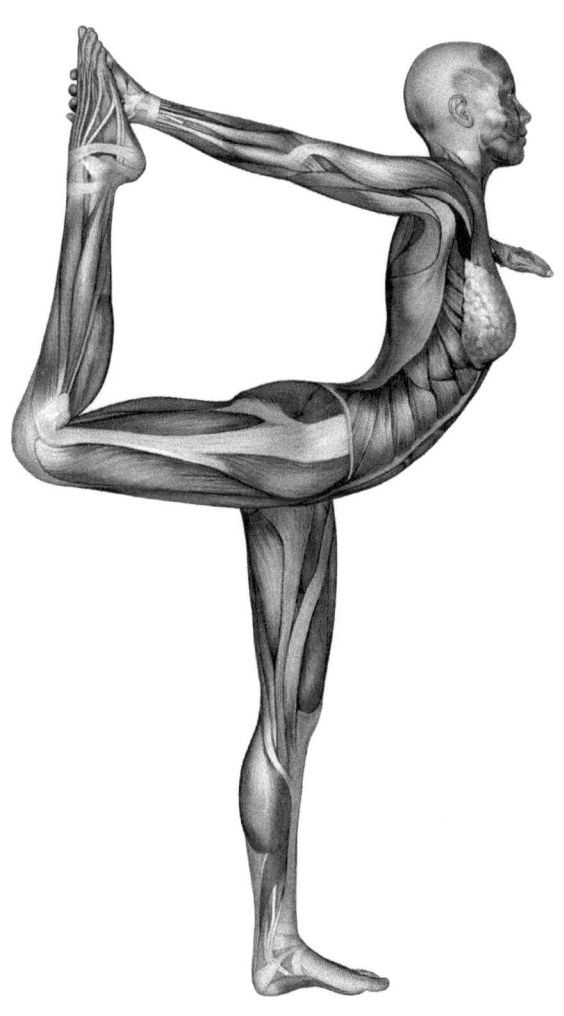

QUEST 1D
MUSCULAR SYSTEM

Observation

Focus your awareness on your physical posture during your daily activities. Often, observing your movements and physical sensations will require you... to... slow... down.

Your muscular system is always communicating with you through its language of internal sensation and postural alignment. If you don't slow down and listen to its whisper, eventually the unpleasant sensations become much more noticeable, communicating with your nervous system in a firm voice of muscular discomfort or a yell of chronic pain.

Action

This week, focus on learning the language of your body. Notice and acknowledge any physical discomfort. Add to your day the simple, gentle daily stretches your body asks for. Consider adding a session of gentle yoga or massage therapy to your weekly schedule. With tender care, physically touch and mentally acknowledge the parts of your muscular system that need attention. As deeper layers of your muscular system wake up and start communicating with your nervous system, new sensations that may be mildly uncomfortable will present themselves and ask for attention. Acknowledge these signals and act mindfully to address them. As with all practices in this book, consider researching the subject more deeply, taking a class, or asking an expert as needed. While the interactions of the muscular system are complex, every step gives an opportunity to mindfully master your muscular understanding and control.

Duration and Frequency

Try to become aware of your posture as often as possible during your daily activities. Get up, move around, and stretch after every 20 to 40 minutes of sitting. Continue any additional daily or weekly physical practices and therapies for one to six weeks or until you start to feel your muscular awareness expanding naturally.

1D

Insight Job

QUEST LOG 1D
DAY ONE

Date:

Areas of discomfort:

Plan of action:

Concepts deserving further study or practice:

Chapter One: Human Body

QUEST LOG 1D
DAY TWO

Date:

Areas of discomfort:

Today's mindful movement activities:

Today's muscular therapy activities:

Areas of improvement or increased awareness:

Focus areas for tomorrow's practice:

Concepts deserving further study or practice:

Week Four: Nervous System

The human nervous system is an incredibly complex network that can have a great impact on your overall health and quality of life. Each breath you take, each beat of your heart, all your voluntary and involuntary movements, and even your digestion all depend on a flawless communication hub between the brain and spinal cord. Your nervous system is responsible for your very basic life functions such as respiration, blood pressure, cardiac activity, and myotatic reflexes. Supporting your nervous system balance is fundamental to promoting your overall health.

Because diverse bodily functions need to be prioritized differently depending on the situation, the nervous system has different components that respond to different stimuli. The most recognizable nervous system responses are "fight or flight" and "rest and repair." Unfortunately, your nervous system is greatly affected by stress and over-activity (mental or physical). With modern society expecting us to be successful in both personal and professional life with limited time and space for education and support, we often find ourselves in a pattern of constant fight-or-flight response that begins to feel normal.

Whether at home or in the workplace, we create an atmosphere of constant stress and anxiety, sacrificing our present peace of mind while chasing the goal of eventual success. Grades at school and performance reviews at work do not account for our quality of sleep, our stress factors, our ability to relax and recharge, or even our clarity of thought. It's no wonder our society's health has taken a backseat to the health of our financial balance sheet. In today's world, the deck is stacked against our nervous system's well-being.

Chapter One: Human Body

Instead of financially preparing your savings for future illnesses, it is important to invest your time and energy in supporting your state of well-being now. This alone can give you the power and clarity to maneuver through life's multifaceted challenges.

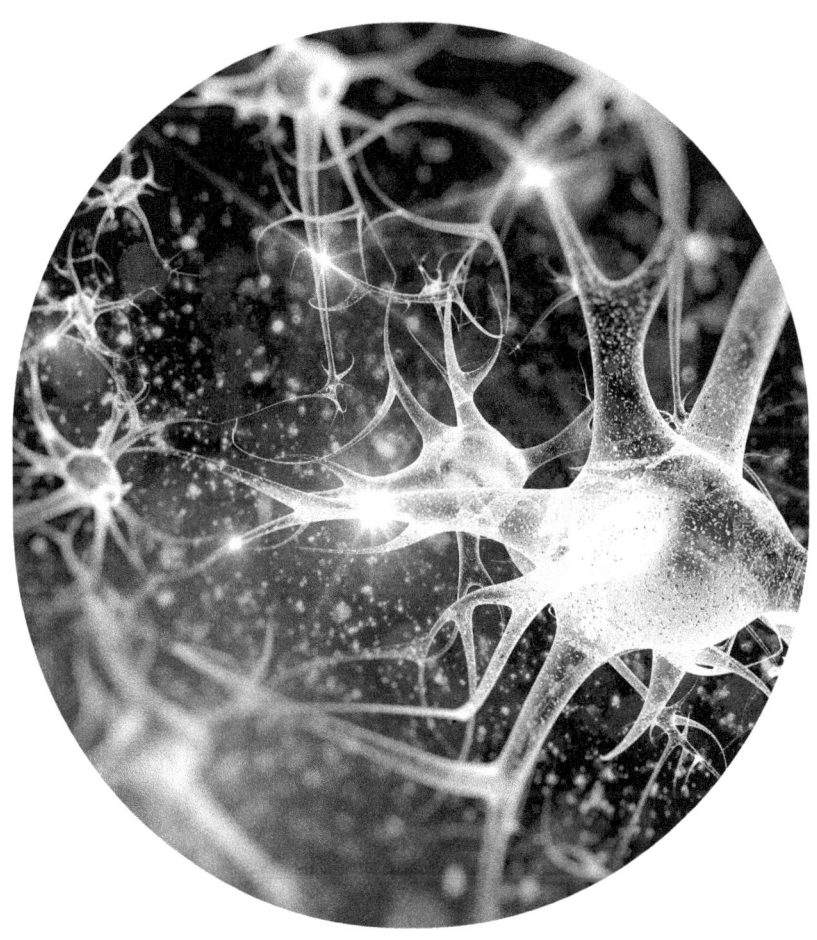

Connected to all other systems, your nervous system never functions alone. It constantly accepts feedback from the furthest reaches of the body and beyond in an attempt to generate an appropriate and well-coordinated response. This response creates both automatic reactions and conscious behavior. As such, it is fitting that the most accessible way to access and modify the current state of the nervous system is through the breath, which we can both observe passively and control consciously. Because it is so closely linked to nervous system response, intimate familiarity with your breath serves as a valuable tool for self-understanding and self-regulation.

As you examine your various breathing patterns, you will better understand how internal and external circumstances affect them. Short, shallow breaths with the inhale lasting longer than the exhale indicates an active fight-or-flight system. Slow, deep breaths with the exhale lasting longer than the inhale, is representative of a calmer nervous system state. Because you have conscious control of your breath, simple breathing exercises are a great place to start when trying to bring balance to the nervous system. To gain better control of your nervous system at any time, learn the 4-7-8 breathing pattern, described below by Dr. Andrew Weil, and apply it whenever needed:

> *The 4-7-8 breathing exercise is utterly simple, takes almost no time, requires no equipment and can be done anywhere. Although you can do the exercise in any position, sit with your back straight while learning the exercise. Place the tip of your tongue against the ridge of tissue just behind your upper front teeth, and keep it there through the entire exercise. You will be exhaling through your mouth around your tongue; try pursing your lips slightly if this seems awkward.*

Chapter One: Human Body

- *Exhale completely through your mouth, making a whoosh sound.*
- *Close your mouth and inhale quietly through your nose to a mental count of four.*
- *Hold your breath for a count of seven.*
- *Exhale completely through your mouth, making a whoosh sound to a count of eight.*
- *This is one breath. Now inhale again and repeat the cycle three more times for a total of four breaths.*

Note that with this breathing technique, you always inhale quietly through your nose and exhale audibly through your mouth. The tip of your tongue stays in position the whole time. Exhalation takes twice as long as inhalation. The absolute time you spend on each phase is not important; the ratio of 4:7:8 is important. If you have trouble holding your breath, speed the exercise up but keep to the ratio of 4:7:8 for the three phases. With practice, you can slow it all down and get used to inhaling and exhaling more and more deeply.

This breathing exercise is a natural tranquilizer for the nervous system. Unlike tranquilizing drugs, which are often effective when you first take them but then lose their power over time, this exercise is subtle when you first try it, but gains in power with repetition and practice. Do it at least twice a day. You cannot do it too frequently. Do not do more than four breaths at one time for the first month of practice. Later, if you wish, you can extend it to eight breaths. If you feel a little lightheaded when you first breathe this way, do not be concerned; it will pass.

Once you develop this technique by practicing it every day, it will be a very useful tool that you will always have with you. Use it whenever anything upsetting happens – before you react. Use it whenever you are aware of internal tension or stress. Use it to help you fall asleep. This exercise cannot be recommended too highly. Everyone can benefit from it.[3]

QUEST 1E
NERVOUS SYSTEM

Observation

This week, you have only one job: taking ownership of your own health. Determine the best approach to support your nervous system. Start by observing your sleep pattern and your mental-emotional state as it changes with different activities throughout the week. Which activities felt draining and which left you feeling recharged? Who was responsible for creating these activities? What factors can you control to increase your level of balance and peace and decrease your level of disturbance and unease?

Action

Add your own peaceful, recharging activities to your week or work with some of the suggestions below, monitoring any changes throughout the week.

- Consume brain foods and supplements that support the nervous system (including omega-3 fatty acids, chamomile tea, and magnesium).
- Increase the quality and quantity of the water you drink.
- Safely and gradually increase your sun exposure.
- Spend time outside or take a walk on a nature trail.

- Practice deep breathing using common yoga or meditation techniques.

Activities that calm the nervous system offer relaxation and reward you with renewed energy to more calmly address the rest of your life's activities. This week, have fun finding and appreciating some time to relax.

Duration and Frequency

Pay attention to the state of your nervous system as often as possible during the day. After observing for some time, begin to practice deep breathing or other stress reduction techniques if you find your nervous system too often in a state of fight-or-flight.

Practice for one to three weeks or until you feel you have a better understanding of the stress triggers in your daily life and your nervous system's response.

Insight Job

QUEST LOG 1E
DAY ONE

Date:

General observations of nervous system status:
(Mental-emotional state, sleep pattern, and other contributing activities)

Activities to add (goal):

Activities to avoid (goal):

Concepts deserving further study or practice:

Chapter One: Human Body

QUEST LOG 1E
DAY TWO

Date: _____

General observations of nervous system status and changes:
_____
_____
_____
_____

Today's balancing activities:
_____
_____
_____
_____

Today's disturbing activities:
_____
_____
_____
_____

Focus areas for tomorrow's practice:
_____
_____
_____

Concepts deserving further study or practice:
_____
_____
_____

Week Five: Immune System

The human immune system is responsible for protecting us from the disease-causing microorganisms, such as bacteria, viruses, and fungi that surround us at all times. Activated before birth (during the second trimester), your immune system protects you for your entire life. It functions throughout the different systems of the body in various forms and adapts in reaction to new or evolving pathogens. Everyone has a unique immune system that responds differently to the diverse range of actual and perceived environmental threats.

Many people enhance their immune system through lifestyle changes, as there are many factors that indirectly affect immune system health. For instance, your personal hygiene, food intake, surrounding environment, sleep quality, and stress levels can all support or weigh on your immune system. Therefore, it can be helpful to mindfully address these areas of your lifestyle to give your immune system its best chance to keep you healthy.

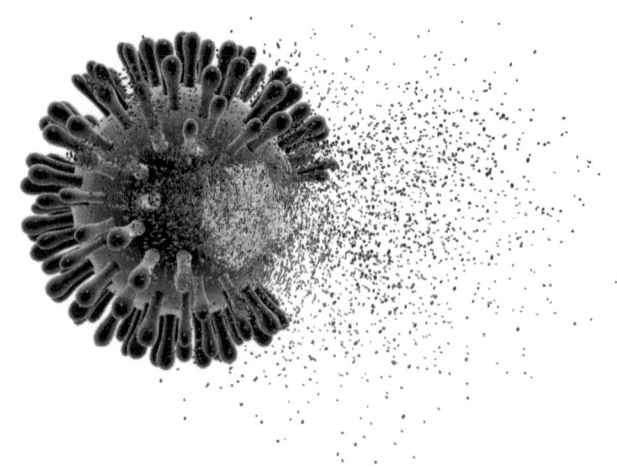

QUEST 1F
IMMUNE SYSTEM

Action

This week, dedicate your energy and attention to a mindful practice of supporting the immune system naturally. Follow the simple steps provided below and do your own research on how the following factors are already affecting your health:

Personal hygiene:

Supporting your immune system can be as easy as protecting it from environmental assaults naturally with a simple hygiene routine such as washing your hands before and after every meal to preventing infections.

Food and micronutrients:

This week, increase your dietary focus. Try to eat more natural, whole foods such as fruits, vegetables, and whole grains (if tolerated well). If eating meat, cook it thoroughly and avoid cross-contamination while preparing food. If you smoke or drink, practice moderation this week. Consider adding some naturally derived supplements or whole foods that contain vitamin C, B-complex, A, and zinc to support your immune system—but consult your physician first.

Surrounding environment:

The more pathogens you take in, the more work your immune system must do. Try to reduce your exposure to pollutants and contaminants. Stay away from sick friends and avoid polluted air as much as possible. Wearing adequate personal protection, thoroughly clean your living space and working environment.

Sleep quality:

Your immune system is a complex mechanism that performs based on your internal clock. Maintaining seven to eight hours of sleep at night on a consistent schedule allows the immune system to perform at its best in terms of defense, support, and recovery.

Psychological stress:

While your immune system is actively responsible for your internal health, you are responsible for the external factors that can affect your immune system. Stress can interfere with your immune system in ways that few can afford. Although you may not be able to control the external world and stressful situations, you can mostly control how you respond to those unpleasant circumstances. Continue taking time this week to recognize stressful situations as they occur, then use some simple stress management tactics to overcome or accept the discomfort these situations cause. Experiment to find out what works best for you.

Chapter One: Human Body

Duration and Frequency

During this practice, focus on the factors that influence your immune system as often as you can recognize them.

Practice for one to three weeks or until you feel your immune system trends toward balance. Listen to your body's signals of health or disease to determine when you're comfortable moving on.

1F

QUEST LOG 1F
DAY ONE

Date:

General observations of immune function & contributing activities:

Personal hygiene goal:

Food and micronutrients goal:

Environment quality goal:

Chapter One: Human Body

QUEST LOG 1F

Sleep goal:

Psychological stress goal:

Concepts deserving further study or practice:

Insight Job

QUEST LOG 1F
DAY TWO

Date:

General observations of immune function & any notable changes:

Personal hygiene goal status:

Food and micronutrients goal status:

Environment quality goal status:

Chapter One: Human Body

QUEST LOG 1F

Sleep goal status:

Psychological stress goal status:

Focus areas for tomorrow's practice:

Concepts deserving further study or practice:

Week Six: Skeletal System

To exist as an advanced organism that can pick itself up and move independently over land, the human body needs a well-defined protective framework. The skeletal system reliably serves these and other needs, and does so in surprisingly active and dynamic ways. Mechanically, it is responsible for providing muscles and connective tissues with places to attach and a structure from which to generate force. (This is especially complex around the spine.) Protective structures, such as the skull, vertebrae, and rib cage, dutifully guard vital organs and communication pathways. The skeleton also stores essential minerals (calcium and phosphorous, among others) and releases them as needed to maintain blood homeostasis. The bones of the skeletal system can recover from injury and are even flexible. Like the muscular system, it doesn't only need the right nutrients, but also requires regular loading and unloading to stay healthy. As the skeletal system works unceasingly to support us in a shape more complex than a puddle, it deserves our mindful support during this week of practice.

Chapter One: Human Body

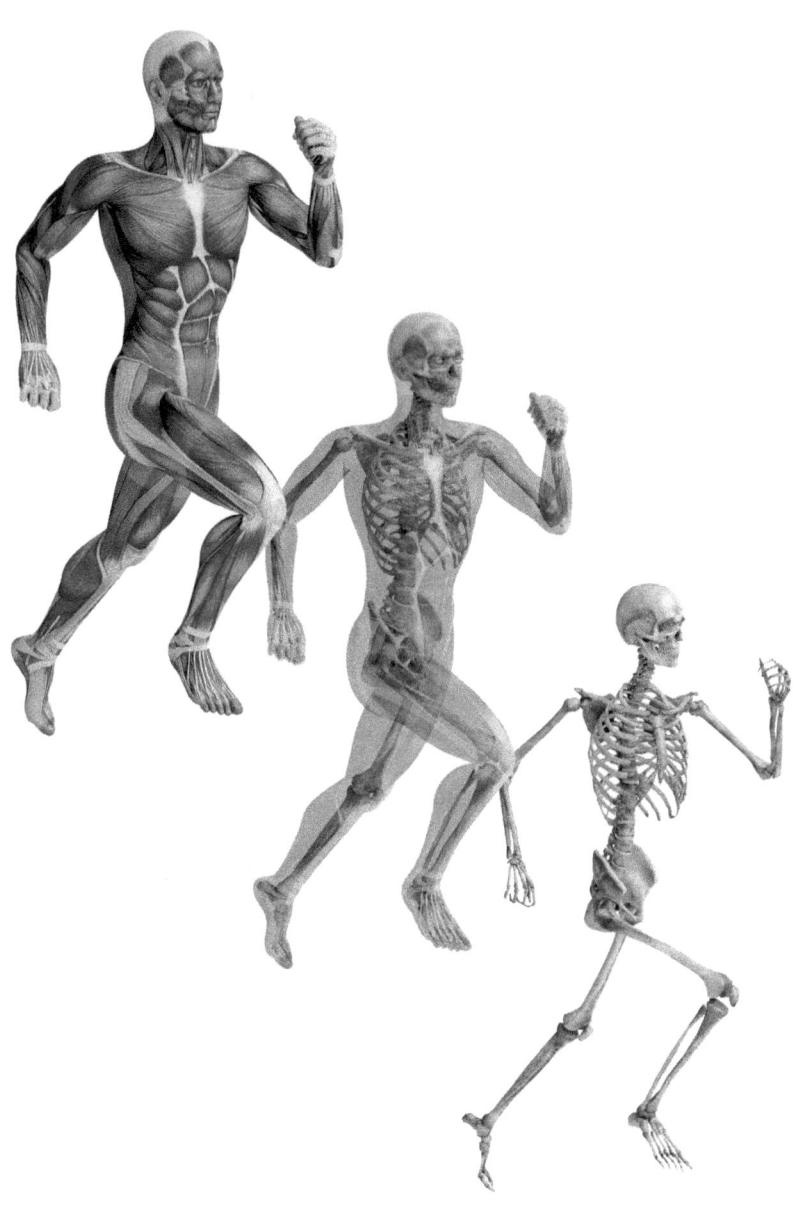

QUEST 1G
SKELETAL SYSTEM

Action

This week, dedicate your energy and attention to a mindful practice of naturally supporting all aspects of the skeletal system. Follow the simple steps provided below and do some research to discover how the following factors are already affecting your health.

Mechanical

Support your skeletal system by aligning your spine. Continue increasing your focus on posture, using simple yoga stretches daily to improve your spinal alignment. Practice spinal movements that activate your spine in all five directions (flexion, extension, lateral flexion, rotation, and axial extension). You could also enjoy a guided self-massage (for the superficial layer of muscles) or visit a qualified, experienced massage therapist to experience the release and increased spinal awareness that deep tissue massage can provide.

Chapter One: Human Body

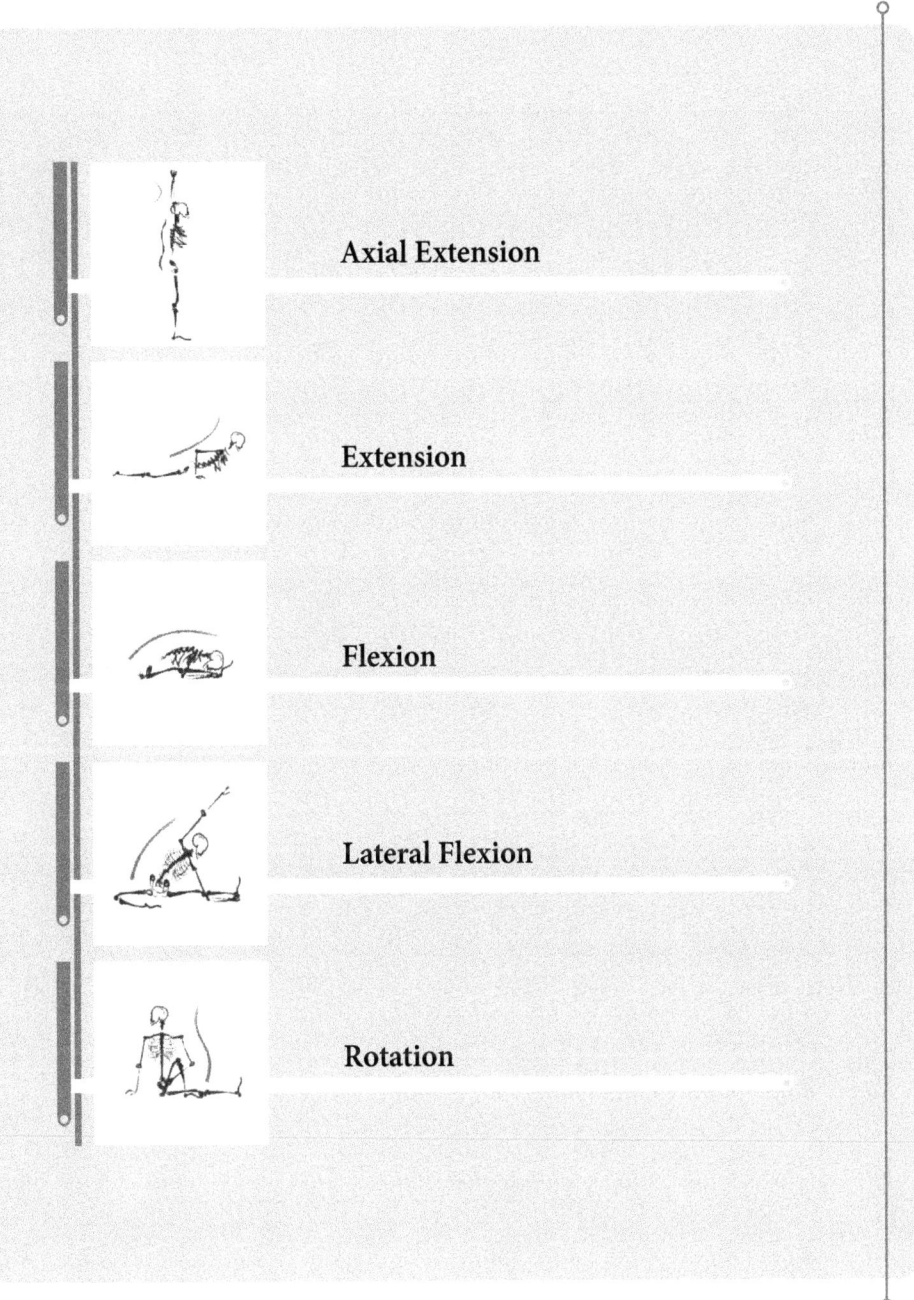

Axial Extension

Extension

Flexion

Lateral Flexion

Rotation

Action (continued)

Protective

Help protect your protective bones from the outside in. Some examples include: using your seatbelt while driving, wearing a helmet while riding a bike ride or playing sports, wearing the proper personal protective equipment at work or when working on projects at home, and generally avoiding harsh physical activities that could injure your skeletal system.

Metabolic

To provide your skeletal system with its essential building blocks, you need to offer your body food that contains skeletal building blocks. Improve your diet by introducing foods or supplements that provide natural sources of calcium, phosphorus, collagen, omega 3 fatty acids, and vitamins D, A, B12, K2, and C.

Duration and Frequency

Focus on the skeletal system for about one week unless you are experiencing bone-related difficulties or have a family history of bone problems. In such cases, now is a good time to do some more research or see a specialist.

Chapter One: Human Body

QUEST LOG 1G
DAY ONE

Date:

General observations of skeletal system function:

Mechanical support goal:

Protective support goal:

Metabolic support goal:

Concepts deserving further study or practice:

Insight Job

QUEST LOG 1G
DAY TWO

Date:

General observations or improvements of skeletal system function:

Mechanical support goal status:

Protective support goal status:

Metabolic support goal status:

Focus areas for tomorrow's practice:

Concepts deserving further study or practice:

Chapter One: Human Body

Week Seven: Endocrine System

By this point, you should be more tuned-in to the messages that your body is sending all the time. The endocrine system, also known as the hormone system, is a network of glands and hormones responsible for sending and modifying many of the important messages communicated between body systems and eventually brought to the attention of our conscious awareness.

Hormones, chemical messengers made by the nine glands of the endocrine system, are released into the bloodstream to communicate with the nervous system and coordinate an appropriate response to stimuli such as growth, reproduction, stress, or injury. Hormones also control many biological processes. For instance, the thyroid gland supports growth, development, and metabolism. Male and female hormones are critical for sexual health and often dictate emotions. Cortisol ("stress hormone"), released by the adrenal gland, communicates with the nervous system and brain to regulate blood pressure, blood sugar, body energy levels, and the fight-or-flight response.

Imbalance in the endocrine system may lead to a range of health problems including anxiety, blood sugar imbalances, diabetes, weight gain, obesity, immune system suppression, heart and blood pressure imbalances, and more.

Insight Job

QUEST 1H
ENDOCRINE SYSTEM

Action

This week our mindfulness practice supports our endocrine system by reducing stress response from the inside out. Long ago, during a meditation retreat, I learned a very powerful practice from a Buddhist monk to help handle the results of stressful situations. I have successfully used this method for almost a decade with restorative and yin yoga practitioners to help them overcome their daily stress. The technique was called "RAIN."

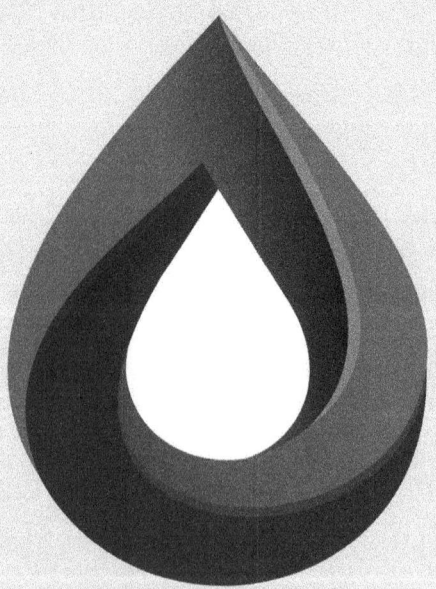

Chapter One: Human Body

R - Recognition

At the end of each day, take a moment to recognize the events and circumstances where you found yourself stressed.

A - Allowance

Once you have listed your recognized stressors, allow yourself to observe your reactions toward those circumstances without further judgment.

I - Identification

After recognition and allowance, identify each stress factor and ask yourself the following questions: *"Why did it make me feel that way?"* *"What can I do about it?"* and *"How could I react to this calmly?"*

N - Nonattachment

Now that you have recognized, allowed, and identified your stress factors for today, remind yourself that you are more than your mind and your emotions. You cannot afford to hold on to those feelings and neither can your endocrine system. There's no need to risk your physical and mental health because of minor stressors.

Let it go, wash it away.

This week, you are invited to practice RAIN to meet and overcome daily stress and anxieties. Some of your stressors may seem insignificant; however, depending on the amount of attention and energy you dedicate to them, your endocrine system may respond to them in major ways. Let's wash it all away with RAIN.

Action (continued)

As an additional technique to support stress response and to help rejuvenate all systems of the body, consider spending this week getting more in touch with your breath. As you may have already discovered when working with the muscular system and nervous system, the focused breath can serve as a very valuable tool to either energize or relax any part of the body and mind. When you are taking full, steady inhales, you may feel a sense of physical strength and mental sharpness. Alternatively, by allowing yourself to exhale fully and by increasing the duration of exhalation, you can generate a sense of relaxation, relief, and calm.

Normally, the breath automatically reacts to signals from other systems of the body. With practice, simply tuning into your current breathing pattern, without manipulation, can provide an expanding wealth of information about your natural response to the current situation. This awareness can even bring physical systems closer to balance without any further effort. Once you become more familiar with the subtleties of your breath, you can even focus your attention on an uncomfortable physical or mental sensation then "breathe it out," exhaling through your mouth, feeling relief as the sensation dissipates.

Work with your breath and the RAIN technique this week to learn how to manage your stress response from the inside out.

Duration and Frequency

Practice RAIN daily at the end of the day for one to three weeks or until you feel you have a better understanding of the main stressors in your life. Mindful breathing and the RAIN technique can also be used any time that you feel the physical, mental, or emotional toll of a stressful situation.

This is the last quest in the chapter. Now is a good time to take stock of any physical stress that has become apparent over the course of the chapter. If you desire to continue your physical development based on a set plan, your Quest Log has space for you to create an Action Plan to carry with you as you move forward. Otherwise, continue working to raise awareness of your health and to maintain your physical form during daily activity. You will soon experience many of the positive changes that a healthier lifestyle can provide.

1H

Insight Job

QUEST LOG 1H
DAY ONE

Date:

Stressors identified and released through RAIN:

Observations on the breath:

Focus areas for tomorrow's practice:

Concepts deserving further study or practice:

Chapter One: Human Body

QUEST LOG 1H
DAY TWO

Date:

Stressors identified and released through RAIN:

Observations on the breath:

Focus areas for tomorrow's practice:

Concepts deserving further study or practice:

Insight Job

QUEST LOG
PHYSICAL ACTION PLAN

Date:

General physical focus areas moving forward:

Integumentary system plan and goals:

Digestive system plan and goals:

Muscular system plan and goals:

Chapter One: Human Body

QUEST LOG

Nervous system plan and goals:

Immune system plan and goals:

Skeletal system plan and goals:

Endocrine system plan and goals:

Concepts to study further:

After practicing the quests in the preceding chapter, you are now reminded of your complex physical body and its needs. At this point, you are a living example of how mindfully maintaining a healthier lifestyle supports your entire state of being. The next chapter focuses on a non-physical aspect of our existence. You are encouraged to continue your simple physical practices to improve your quality of your life, day by day.

Because you committed to your own physical health improvement, now you are responsibly conscious of your body from a higher perspective than before. Next, you will work to responsibly connect with your mental state.

Every belief system (spiritual, mechanical, philosophical, medical, etc.) introduces a psychological framework or paradigm to *define, direct,* and *discipline* human nature, the meaning of life, and life's purpose. It is through that worldview that we, as human beings, create a coherent picture of reality for ourselves, our communities, and our society. Our living standards, intentions, choices, and actions create our reality frame for ourselves and others, whether we are fully conscious of it or not.

In the following chapter, you begin a mindful practice to improve your mental health and emotional stability. You're not trying to create a paradigm shift nor manipulate your current belief system, but rather use simple techniques to improve your current experience. The simple practice of contemplation, analysis, and understanding of your daily mental activities is just as important, valuable, and effective as your physical health care. Through this mental observation, you can enhance your current state of awareness to greater heights of understanding and compassion.

Chapter One: Human Body

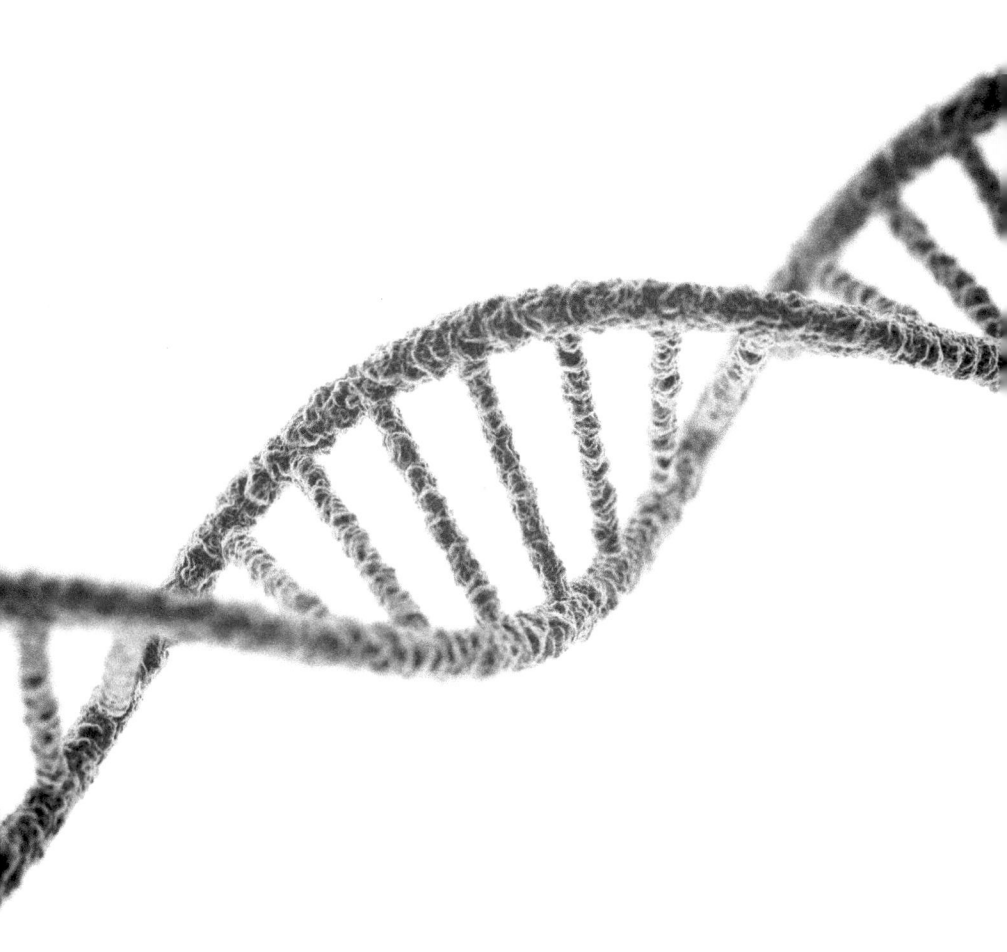

End of Chapter One

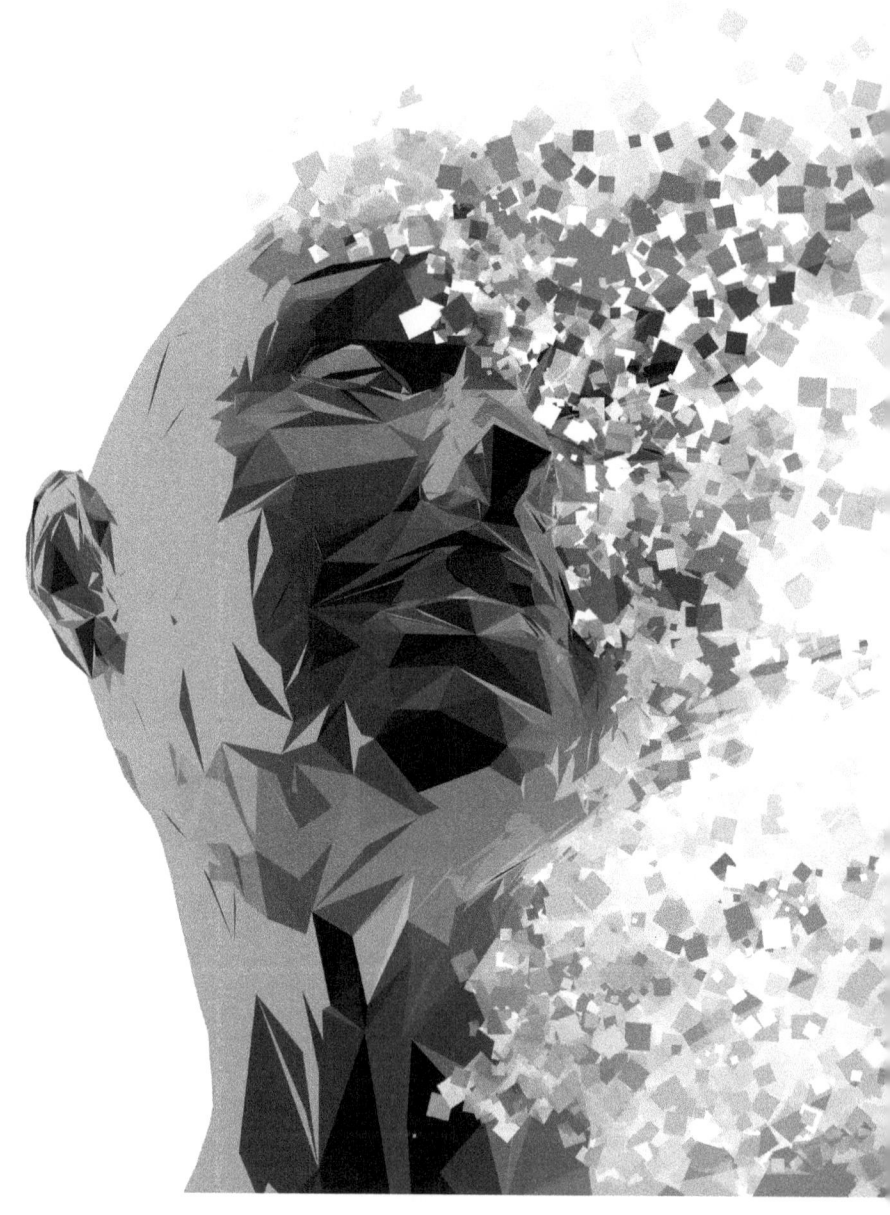

Chapter Two

HUMAN MIND

IN CHAPTER ONE you began your journey within, exploring the realms of mindful practices for your body. After creating your own practices and executing them, you have now begun to feel the benefits of increased awareness and improved well-being of the physical form. Hopefully you found that, in today's world, working with your physical state is easier than ever. Thanks to our scientific and technological development, there is very little argument on the existence of our human body systems and the effect they have on our overall health. Information (occasionally contradictory, but often consistent) about exercise, nutrition, and supplementation is easily accessible locally and online. You probably found that your heightened awareness of your own body was helpful in filtering this material to implement the practices that are best suited for you.

On the other hand, the "non-physical" state of the human being, including our mental, emotional, and spiritual connections and health, has yet to be fully accepted, understood, and agreed upon by the scientific community. As our scientific instruments are not adept at detecting and measuring non-physical parameters (such as emotion, sensation, thought, intuition, and other relatively etheric phenomena), and because of the complex, invisible nature of non-physical interactions, objective study of the non-physical human form remains difficult. Brain imagining technology, the study of our body's electromagnetic field, and quantum physics are beginning to shed light on this previously unseen reality; but, for now, science and spirituality/philosophy exist as largely separate fields of study.

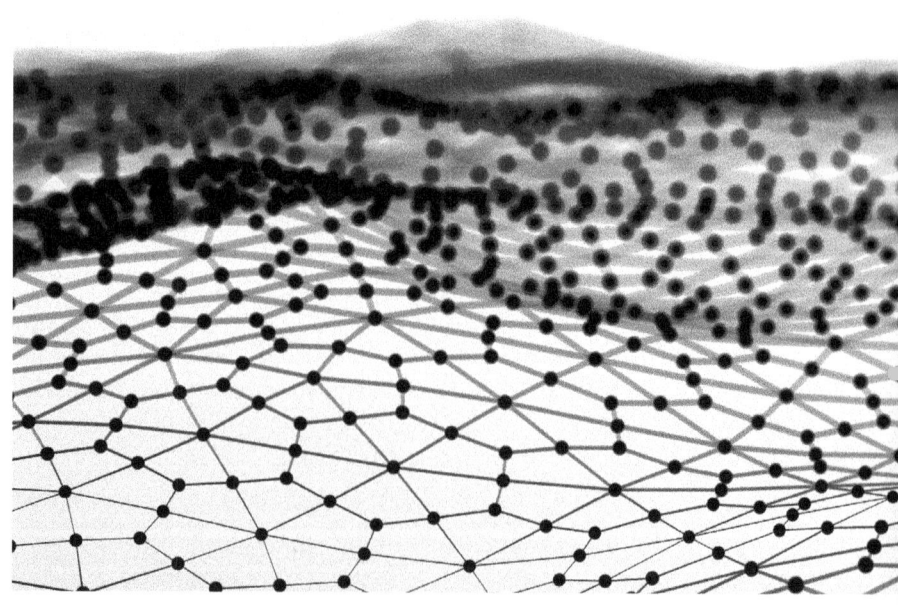

Chapter Two: Human Mind

Fortunately, human beings are born equipped with the ability to expand awareness of the non-physical body from the inside out. In this chapter, you will work to extend your own awareness beyond the limits of external instrumentation. By investigating within your own being, you can discover and understand more about yourself than anything or anyone outside yourself can tell you. During the following weeks, you will explore the human mind and its reactions to physical and non-physical stimuli. The goal of these practices is to make you aware of your own states of mind by *consciously* observing the mind's fluctuations. After we build a foundational understanding of the mind through Chapter Two, we will expand our awareness to deeper portions of our non-physical existence throughout Chapters Three and Four, as well as in subsequent books.

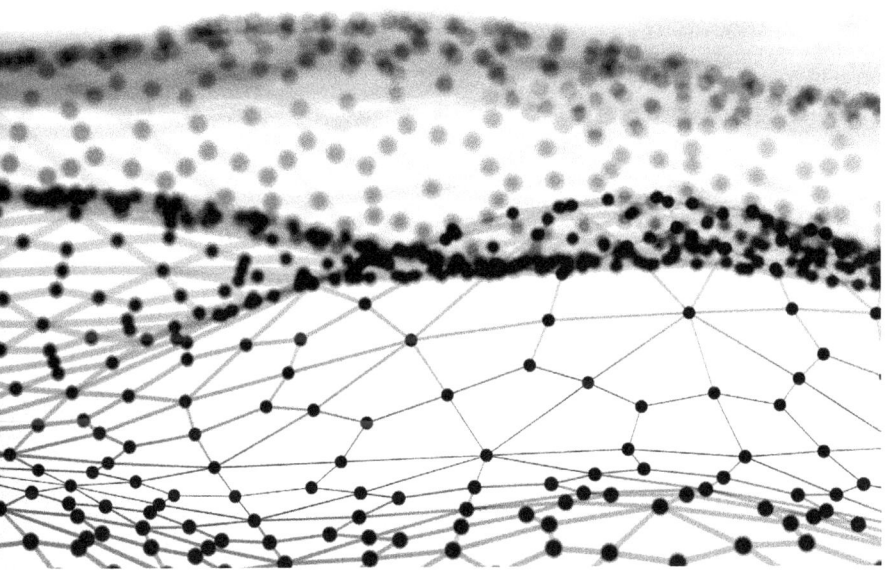

QUEST 2A
WHAT DO I KNOW?

Fittingly, to comprehend the nature of the human mind, you must both open your mind and go beyond your mind. We all understand there are countless possible physical experiences for our bodies. Similarly, it is important to accept the reality of infinite, equally complex realms of non-physical experience for our minds. (Consider the familiar states of elation, depression, rumination, imagination, and dream.)

The first quest of this chapter is the simple observation of your current awareness and understanding of the human mind. Most people have never considered the complexity of the mind, so there is no need for judgment during this practice. Do not overthink or research externally in search of validation. This practice displays that which your mind has already registered within itself. It displays how you mentally perceive the world around you, including yourself. Depending on your life experiences, this perception could be totally or partially psychological, rational, emotional, or spiritual. Take the next 15 to 20 minutes to complete the exercise below before continuing further into Chapter Two.

Observation

Briefly review the diagram on the facing page, then ask yourself the questions that follow.

Chapter Two: Human Mind

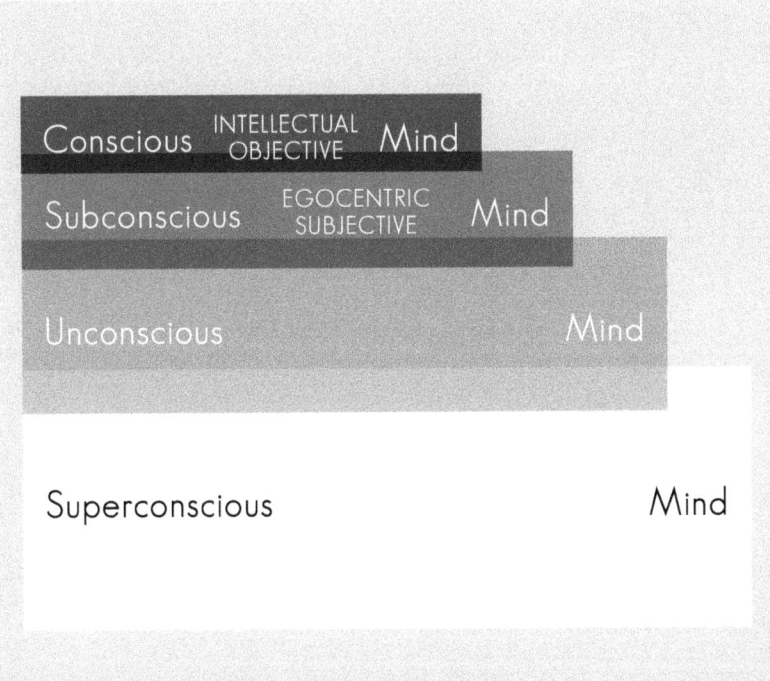

Who am I?

What am I doing?

Why and how am I doing this?

Duration and Frequency

Experience this observation only once for as long as it takes to understand your current perception of the mind. Record this in your Quest Log.

2A

QUEST LOG 2A
WHO AM I?

Date:

Who am I? What am I doing? Why and how am I doing this?

Summary of my current perception of the mind:

Chapter Two: Human Mind

QUEST LOG 2A

My current definition of conscious mind:

My current definition of subconscious mind:

My current definition of unconscious mind:

My current definition of superconscious mind:

QUEST 2B
CULTIVATE A LITTLE MINDFULNESS

Now that you have reviewed your current level of awareness of the human mind and its relation to your life experiences, it is time to expand your understanding from within by focusing your attention on the unique nature of each layer of the mind. This chapter presents mental activities in the same format as the physical body practices. Each week you will explore a deeper layer of the mind to build your understanding from within. Similar to your experience with the physical body, your first quest is to simply take stock of your current state of mental health.

You have planted the seed for your Tree of Life seed by diligently expanding awareness of the physical body. Now you will focus on different states of mental health that allow that seed to grow. You understand that you are more than skin, muscles, bones, nerves, and hormones; you exist as a product of the interrelated functions of all body systems working in harmony. You may already be reaping some of the benefits that this more spacious sense of self can bring to your experience of life.

Continuing your expansion toward full integration of the human form, it is fitting to begin a daily practice focused on cultivating awareness of the mental framework that informs your bodily actions. In the following practice, you will explore and document the nutrients that you currently feed your Tree of Life.

Observation

Start by finding yourself a comfortable place to sit and relax. It would be best to pick the same location for these daily activities. Once seated, simply observe your current mental activities. Observe your emotions, thoughts, feelings, and any internal or external sounds and sensations. In this state, your goal is to observe as much as possible and gather information about your current mental state of being. You could observe repeating thought patterns and even the stimulations that cause the mind to generate more thoughts (such as sounds, sensations, or other thoughts). Your goal is just to observe without any judgment or manipulation.

Duration and Frequency

This quest could take 15 to 30 minutes and should be practiced daily until you are familiar with your thought patterns. When comfortable, begin practicing the next quest in this chapter after completing the first day of this quest.

2B

Insight Job

QUEST LOG 2B
DAY ONE

Date:

Main thoughts:

Emotions and feelings:

Sounds or stimulations:

Overall mental state and any other observations:

Chapter Two: Human Mind

QUEST LOG 2B
DAY TWO

Date:

Main thoughts:

Emotions and feelings:

Sounds or stimulations:

Overall mental state and any other observations:

Insight Job

Week One: Conscious Mind

Your conscious mind is the layer of the intellectual mind that you are aware of and work with objectively. It is where you collect novel information from all senses and generate thoughts for analysis and decision making. The state of your conscious mind defines your ability to focus on a single matter and solve problems. As such, this layer is where you learn to explore and expand concentration techniques. This is the most commonly known layer of the mind, simply because of its importance for mental tasks and professional responsibilities. Unfortunately, that is also why this layer of mind is often overworked and occasionally abused.

Imagine owning an advanced computer or generator. One day you decided to turn in on and set it to maximum output, and then never turn it off again, even for maintenance. If the machine were designed properly, then you would expect its self-protection mechanisms to shield it from overwork. In the best case, those mechanisms will protect the computer by slowing it down, reducing power, or rejecting input. Without relief, the machine's output may become inaccurate or improper as it loses its ability to perform at peak capacity. In this state, the machine would no longer appear capable of performing its duties. Knowing the story, we see that the computer has the ability to perform to its highest promised potential, but misuse and the lack of maintenance have exhausted its envisioned abilities.

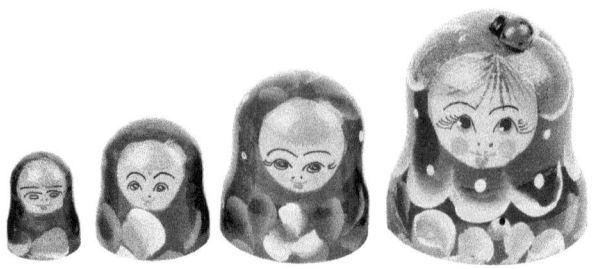

Chapter Two: Human Mind

The human conscious mind in childhood is an advanced mind. As we mature, in addition to growing the distractive habit of "multitasking" (which reduces the machine's efficiency through a constant switching of gears), we can begin to lose or forget our advanced mental abilities. The conscious mind's required maintenance includes concentration, positive contemplation, free creativity, and critical thinking. Without being renewed by these activities, the conscious mind can no longer experience the full spectrum of awareness that it once did. Though we enjoyed this fuller, deeper conscious experience as children, it has since been filtered by other layers of the mind and their (often inadvertently) activated protection mechanisms. Fortunately, you have within you the ability to return your conscious mind to balance, once again experiencing the state of childlike wonder, spontaneity, and expressiveness. The practices in this chapter support both the maintenance of your mental machine and the resting of its protection mechanisms.

To begin rejuvenating your conscious mind and to reward yourself for traveling the path you faced in Chapter One, you are welcomed to practice the following activity for at least a week.

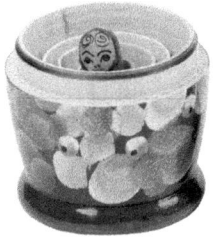

QUEST 2C
CONSCIOUS MIND

Observation

On the first day of this week's quest, begin by spending at least 20 minutes contemplating your favorite activities: those you have truly enjoyed throughout your life and those you want to pursue more deeply. These are the types of activities that involve your attention such that you normally cannot combine them with other activities. Your actions during these activities should require your full concentration, demanding innovation and intellectual involvement. These activities could include reading books, researching a subject of interest, writing, coloring, painting, sculpting, cooking, playing an instrument, singing, woodworking, creating with building toys, manual or computer-aided design, or playing chess and other concentration games—anything you enjoy that holds your attention and interest. If you find yourself interested in learning something new, then you are welcome to consider that subject, too.

List all relevant activities in your Quest Log. Do not list activities that you use to distract yourself from life but do not deeply enjoy.

Chapter Two: Human Mind

Action

After listing your favorite activities in your Quest Log, choose one that can maintain your focus for at least 20 minutes every day. Set aside this time then participate in your chosen activity every day.

Unlike other practice methods, focus on the *quantity* of your practice more than the quality of it. Let yourself enjoy your practice entirely and repeat it daily without focusing on the results or product of your work. Consistency is the key to this quest. Your mind is programmed to achieve its highest quality of concentration by repeating a focus-based activity over and over again. Try to stick with the same activity through the whole week unless you find that you begin "going through the motions" instead of focusing deeply.

You don't have to share the result of your daily activity with anyone else. There is no audience or judgment involved. However, if you are curious about your concentration progress, you may review your dated daily practice record—but only after you have spent at least a week on this quest.

Duration and Frequency

Participate in your chosen activity for at least 20 minutes and continue for as long as you can maintain focus, up to two hours.

Practice once a day for at least one week and up to two weeks.

2C

Insight Job

QUEST LOG 2C
DAY ONE

Date:

List of enjoyable activities:

Selected activity for this week's practice:

Chapter Two: Human Mind

QUEST LOG 2C
DAY TWO

Date:

Today's activity log:

Focus of tomorrow's practice:

Concepts deserving further study or practice:

Week Two: Subconscious Mind

The layer of mind beneath the surface of the conscious mind is the subconscious mind with which you work subjectively. Considered the *unaware* mind, this permanent memory bank quietly records external information primarily from the last trimester of pregnancy through the first six to seven years of life. Your subconscious is the generator of your behaviors and the non-physical realms of *human* experience, as well as the manufacturer of human perception (belief-system) through stimulus-response programs.

Due to the complexity of the subconscious mind, it has been very difficult to utilize or even explain the magnitude of its capacity and operational dimensions. Bruce Lipton, developmental biologist and former researcher at Stanford University's School of Medicine, explains the layer of subconscious mind this way:

> *Unfortunately, the downloaded programs comprising the subconscious data base are derived from recording the behavior of others (parents, siblings and community). ... [And] psychology reveals up to 70% of these "learned" behaviors are disempowering, self-sabotaging and limiting. As importantly, these programmed behaviors are expressed as "energy" vibrations that are not contained in your head. The brain's activity can be read using magnetoencephalograph (MEG) technology, similar to EEG except the probe for MEG readings is outside of the head. Simply your thoughts are not contained in your head but are broadcast into the field.*[4]

Chapter Two: Human Mind

Therefore, your subconscious mind is both the foundation and the association component of your perception and worldview. Through the subconscious mind, you form and define your self-image (ego and superego), establish a relationship with the world around you, and build a direct or indirect connection with a higher power (Supreme Consciousness, The Divine). As mentioned before, this book is not trying to manipulate your current physical or mental state of being, but rather re-fine your human experience as a multidimensional being to allow you to understand how you are already being affected on every level. The goal is to polish our existing worldview, clearing the mind and body from destructive elements that influence our view and generate a false perception (illusion) of reality. In this practice of mental detoxification, we explore interrelated methods to access both the subconscious mind and the conscious mind.

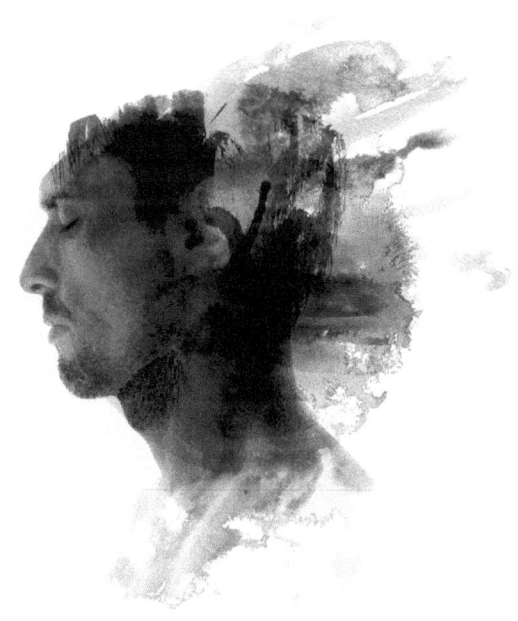

QUEST 2D
SUBCONSCIOUS MIND

This week we will expand upon the RAIN exercise used in the seventh week of Chapter One. RAIN is a great practice to directly work with the objective mind and subjective mind. It allows you to expand your ability to focus on collecting information in an accurate pattern, analyze the thoughts, and decide how to "close the window of an open task" in the mental screening process so that you don't overthink or drain yourself mentally.

Caution: The following practice is designed to help you explore the operations of your conscious and subconscious mind for 20 to 30 minutes daily. Expanding the time and period of this practice without an expert guidance is not recommended and could create addictive overthinking behavior or mental traps.

Observation and Action

Start by finding yourself a comfortable place to sit and relax. Begin by observing your thoughts. If eyes are closed during this practice, the mind usually increases its speed to generate even more thoughts. This is the nature of human mind, to collect information and develop an analysis process. Therefore, when eyes are closed, the human mind slowly disconnects from the world outside and reconnects to the world within. To begin, imagine your conscious mind as a calm and quiet ocean. As you allow your mind to naturally generate thoughts, recognize the thoughts as shorter or longer waves arising on the surface of this ocean. Observe the emotions, thoughts, feelings, sounds, and sensations; then begin to identify and categorize the thoughts.

Thought, emotion, and feeling can normally be categorized as follows:

1. Judgment of present moment, feelings, or sensations

2. Reflection/memory of the past or dream state (can contain happiness, joy, fear, regret, anger, judgment, etc.)

3. Projection of the future (can contain expectations, anxiety, fear, excitement, etc.)

4. Timeless imagination or wandering

5. Observation or analysis of current thought flow

Once you have recognized and identified the current thought allow the wave to pass through your mind without fighting against it or welcoming further expansion. Begin to detach yourself from that thought and redirect your awareness to the clear ocean of your calm mind. In this practice, your mind desires to hold on to each thought, so getting your awareness fully involved is completely normal. Remember that you are neither the conscious nor the subconscious mind alone. The responsibility of these layers of the mind is to collect information from the world outside to be calibrated by the operator. Remind yourself that you are both observer and operator.

In summary, this exercise involves observing thoughts from the sub-conscious layer, letting them come to the conscious surface, collecting and categorizing them, and finally detaching yourself from each thought and moving on.

Recognition,

Allowance,

Identification,

Nonattachment (Nonjudgment)

Note: While practicing RAIN for mental cleansing, you might experience a mental purge. You may be exposed to the pain or pleasure of your own suppressed memories as well as harsh feelings, flashbacks, delusion, fantasy, and both comfortable and uncomfortable mental images. You could become aware of an existing obsession with mental debates or addictive behavior. If you are practicing RAIN properly, then with practice your skills of non-attachment and non-judgment will protect you from the dangers of delusion (identifying yourself with these toxins).

Continue your practice to successfully re-connect the programming and communication pathways between the conscious and subconscious minds. Bruce Lipton elaborates on this process as follows:

Chapter Two: Human Mind

The two minds learn differently. The conscious mind is called creative and can learn by reading a self-help book or going to a lecture, watching a video, or reading an article. It is creative, it goes, 'ah, I have an idea, now I change my mind.' The subconscious mind is a habit mind. And the most important thing about a habit mind is that you don't want it to change very quickly because otherwise, habits fall apart. So it is resistant to change. That is the first thing we have to realize. It is not as easy to change like the creative mind. So how do I change my subconscious mind? How does it learn?

Number one: The first seven years the mind is operating in a low vibrational frequency like hypnosis. So that is one way of changing the program.

Number two: After you are seven you form habits by repeating something over and over and over again. Practicing, repeating, and practicing.

An example: If you read a self-help book the conscious mind understood it, but the subconscious mind learned nothing from it, because you only read it once and this is not how it learns. If you repeat the message of the book over and over and over again and behave that way, then the subconscious mind will learn a new behavior. So it is about habituation, where you make a practice out of something, every day repeat it over and over again.

Duration and Frequency

Practice for at least 20 minutes, but no longer than 30 minutes every day. Practicing longer without expert guidance risks creating additional addictive overthinking patterns.

Practice every day for at least one week and no longer than two weeks.

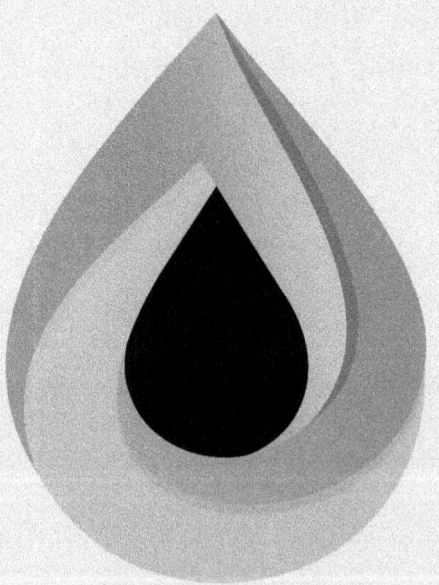

QUEST LOG 2D

DAY ONE

Date:

Overall perception of today's RAIN experience:

Concepts deserving further study or practice:

Chapter Two: Human Mind

QUEST LOG 2D
DAY TWO

Date:

Overall perception of today's RAIN experience:

Concepts deserving further study or practice:

Week Three: Unconscious Mind

The unconscious mind is the most intricate and fascinating layer of the human mind. This layer has intrigued humans for millennia, sparking the creation of profound expression, art, and culture. The human desire to establish a direct relationship with the unconscious mind has inspired the development of countless spiritual disciplines, mystical practices, and esoteric scientific pursuits. The founder of psychoanalysis, Sigmund Freud, introduced us to the soft science of our powerful unconscious mind and its influence on behavior and human interaction with the world. We're now aware of the existence of this layer of the mind that could be defined as the "conditioned foundation" of our psyche. Carl Jung's cognitive psychology provides the basic knowledge of the functionality of the unconscious mind. Through this level of analysis, we have gained a general understanding of the layers of human mind as well as the mind's relation to social perception (archetypes, persona, etc.).

Recently, technology has allowed study of the unconscious mind to evolve into the hard science of neuroscience, granting us the ability to observe and measure the communication of human brainwaves and mental activities. Observation of the information collected by our subconscious mind and conscious mind (riding communication pathways through the unconscious mind) explains the way our mind programs our desires, behaviors, and perception. Consider the adjacent chart, showing a high-level overview of the waveforms generated by different states of mind.

It is no longer a myth that your perception (a byproduct of your unconscious and subconscious mind) shapes your reality, as neuroscience provides us an objective view on this phenomenon.

Chapter Two: Human Mind

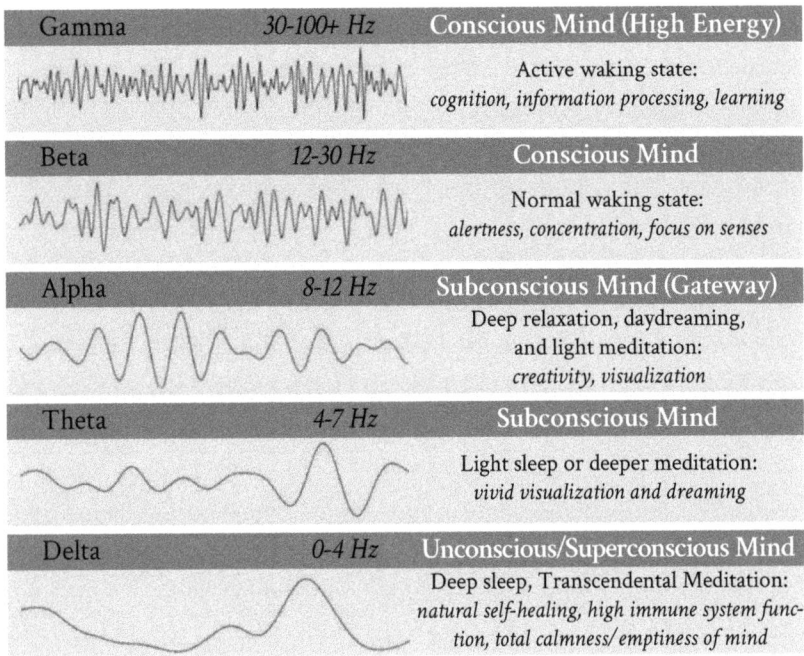

For instance, computer scientists at Google have partnered with neuroscientists to create an artificial neural network, named Deep Dream, that can understand the subtle characteristics and artistic style of images well enough to recreate any other image using the same style. Fascinatingly, if you train this network with one hundred pictures of different breeds of dog then provide it your family portrait, it will return the portrait as a family of dogs, one of which looks suspiciously like your uncle. Alternatively, if you initially input one hundred works by Picasso, your family portrait would be returned as a beautiful cubist masterpiece. The neural network can identify and recreate only what it has been trained to see, whether that identification is objectively valid or not. With all human experience existing as a neural construct, who can state definitively whether your family is a collection of dogs or a masterpiece? How will you define this for yourself?

We see now that these three layers of the mind affect perception. Your unconscious mind is responsible for the formation of a perception-based reality. It connects, processes, and unifies information collected from the subconscious mind. Through this process, the unconscious mind creates a conscious behavior based on your experiences, expectations, desires, and belief system.

While all layers of the mind operate together to present us with our normal state of awareness, the unconscious mind alone connects us to intuition and dreams, both of which are highly valued in ancient cultures and spiritual practices. This week, we will work with these phenomena to explore the mystery of the deeper self.

Chapter Two: Human Mind

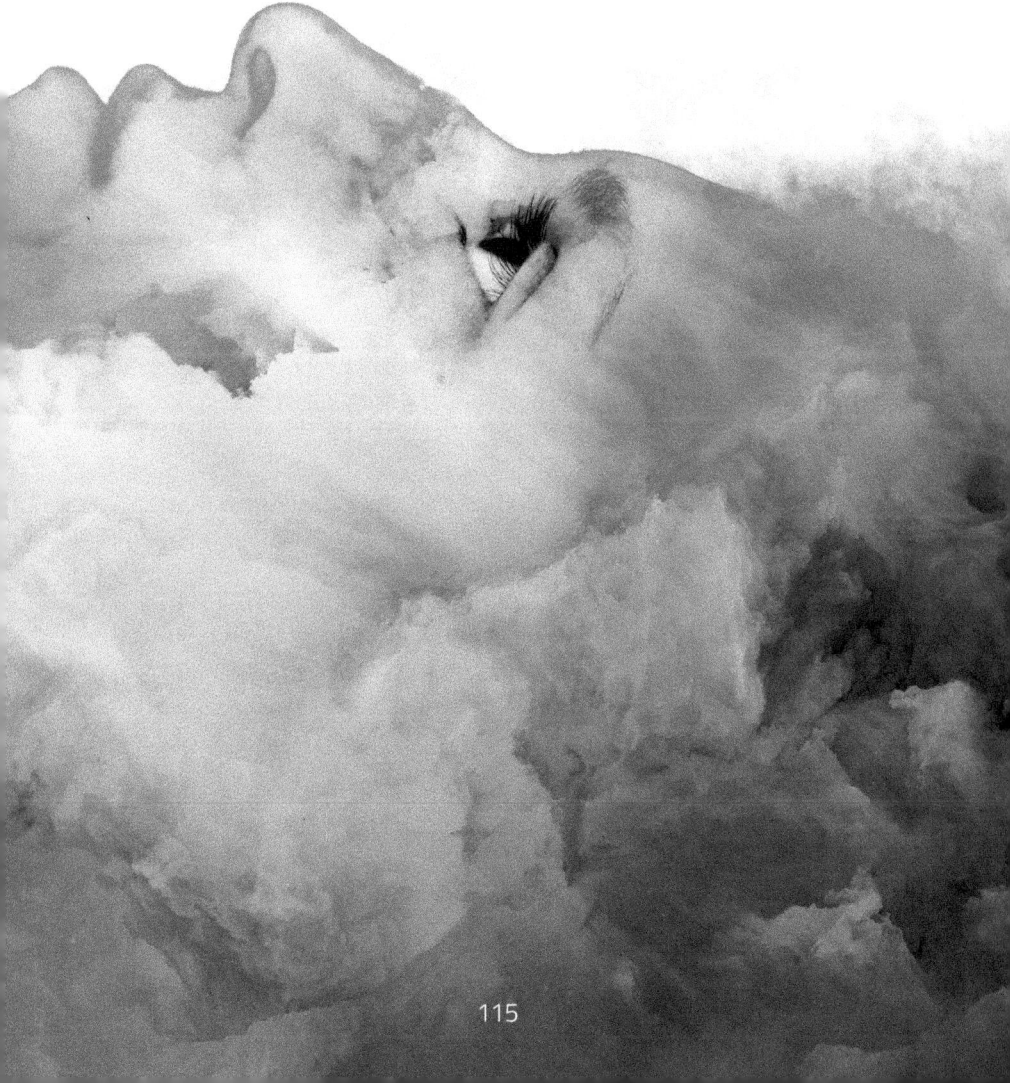

QUEST 2E
UNCONSCIOUS MIND

Observation

This quest empowers your unconscious mind by working with your intuition and acknowledging the content of your dreams.

To begin this practice, you're expected to have a daily exercise of reducing compulsive thinking. To get through to a deeper layer of the mind, you must quiet the other layers first. To accomplish this, dedicate 20 to 30 minutes daily to spend time in nature. After choosing a peaceful location, simply walk or sit and observe the world around you (including the sight of flowers and trees, the sound of wind, birds, rain, and more). No judgment or classification by the mind is required, only pure awareness of the sound, sight, and sensation provided by nature to you.

This week, start a dream/intuition journal and write down any dreams you can remember immediately after waking up. Furthermore, for the daily decisions you make throughout this week, try to let yourself be guided more by your inner voice rather than by hard logic and reason. If you are already involved with any other form of practice to connect with your intuition, now is a good time to enhance or record your daily practice.

Chapter Two: Human Mind

Duration and Frequency

Begin your day with your dream journal, writing your dream descriptions as thoroughly as possible. Then at some point during the day spend at least twenty minutes and up to two hours in nature.

Repeat these exercises every day, without judgment, for one to two weeks.

2E

Insight Job

QUEST LOG 2E
DAY ONE

Date:

Last night's dreams:

Today's nature experience:

Other noteworthy intuitive experiences:

Concepts deserving further study or practice:

Chapter Two: Human Mind

QUEST LOG 2E
DAY TWO

Date:

Last night's dreams:

Today's nature experience:

Other noteworthy intuitive experiences:

Concepts deserving further study or practice:

Insight Job

End of Chapter Two

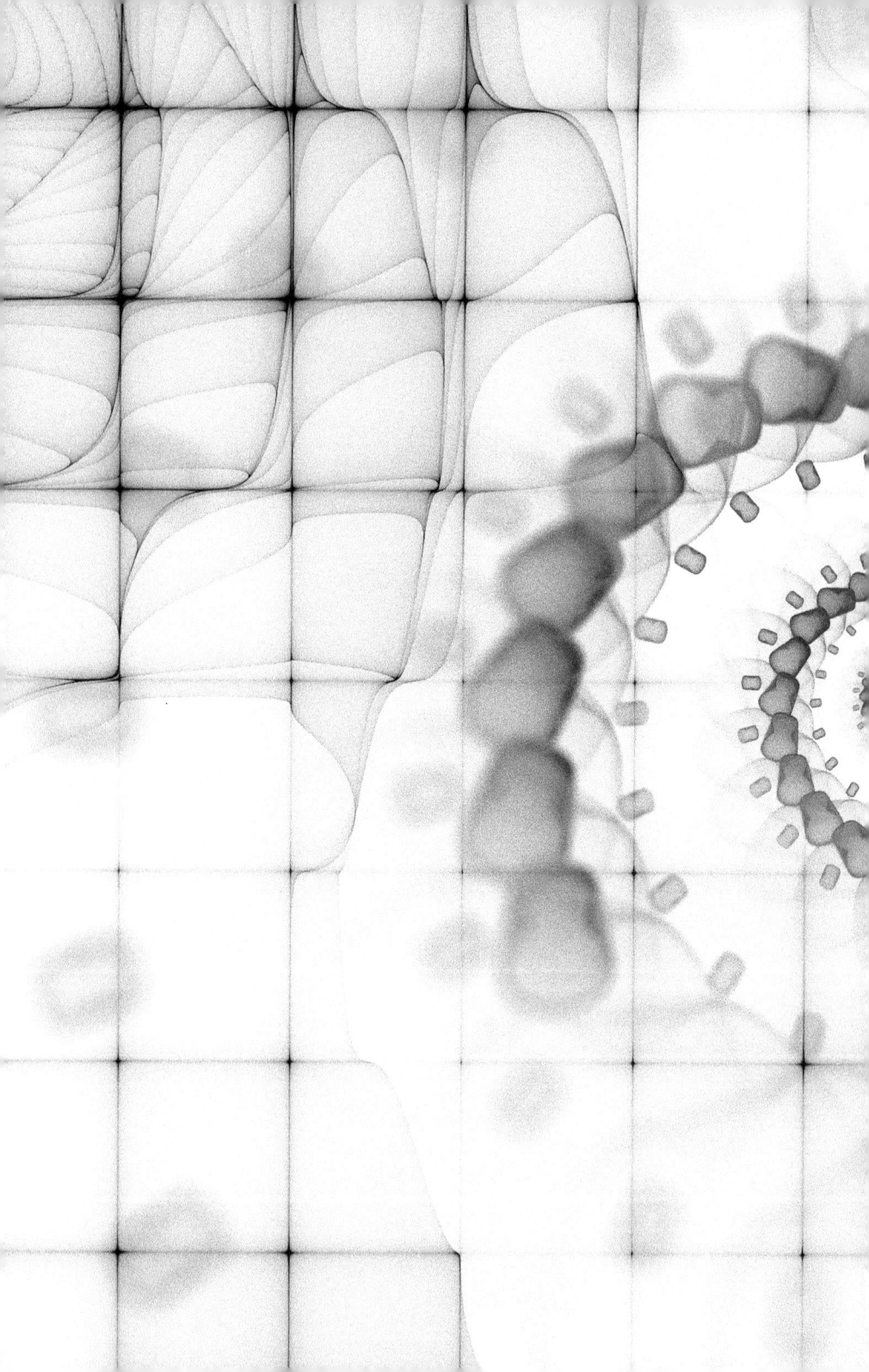

Chapter Three

HUMAN CONSCIOUSNESS

BOTH SPIRITUALITY AND SCIENCE confirm that our convoluted universe has been created by a higher force either purposefully or accidentally. As this force imbues us with awareness, it follows that the force itself possesses a higher level of awareness that may, voluntarily or involuntarily, influence the lower levels, such as the human psyche. Concurrently, the human psyche, both in individual and social settings, yearns to connect to a higher power. When this human desire is linked to what may be considered a higher power, a collective perception is created. This shared perception creates a social reality within the minds and interactions of the population.

This is exactly why the leaders of many ancient cultures and masters of spiritual practices have formed techniques and teachings (including personal and universal ethics) to elevate the individual and shared level of awareness into a higher state, maintaining a cohesive realm of reality for themselves and others using prayers, meditation, and contemplation/concentration techniques. The united practice of the group clarifies the perspective of each individual and unifies the shared perception (social reality), elevating the entire group to a higher level of awareness, communication, and integration of consciousness.

Because the super-conscious mind (i.e., consciousness) is omnipresent, existing beyond the conditions of time and space without limitation, it is impossible to fully comprehend its nature through the linear thought process of the human mind. Understanding of the super-conscious mind is gained only from direct internal experience. Though the super-conscious mind permeates us all, certain noteworthy individuals throughout history (including prophets, sages, and spiritual masters of all types) have been especially talented (gifted) in interpreting and translating the information of the super-conscious mind into teachings relevant to others.

Scientifically, the study of quantum mechanics provides the closest link to describing the relationship between human mind and consciousness. Whether you choose to expand your study or experience of this concept or not, know that your current experiential realm of reality is but one frame of view existing as part of an infinite set of frames throughout space-time. To genuinely expand awareness of your own mind (frame of view), you need to understand the relation between your mind, other minds, and even other forms of consciousness.

Quantum physics and neuroscience congruently propose a theory of higher dimensional interactions with mind and matter. This mental field combines the subjective mind and objective matter to create a higher realm of reality that we call the field of consciousness. The relationship between mind and brain can either increase or decrease the domain of personal reality. In other words, expanding our field of consciousness affects our fundamental understanding of self and the world around us.

Chapter Three: Human Consciousness

Your brain constantly collects and calibrates itself to external and internal input, then re-creates this input as an internal sensation, based not only on the stimulus but also expectations and previous mental models. In neuroscience, the binding problem is the unanswered question of how the human brain cohesively combines—or binds—disparate perceptions (sights, sounds, feelings, and other sensation) of the external world, gathered cooperatively by various parts of the body and processed separately in different parts of the brain, to create a unified perception almost instantaneously. What you consciously experience at any moment is the result of this mysterious process.

Perhaps the closest physical model to demonstrate the consciousness field and the relation between human mind, brain, and information is found in the observation of black holes. Just as the human mind seems to draw in information, the strong attractive force of gravity causes a black hole to collect matter from external space. We cannot see the black hole itself, as light cannot escape its gravity; however, its properties can be inferred from its effect on nearby matter. For instance, a star that wanders too close to a black hole will be pulled apart by the gravity, emitting high-energy x-rays that can be detected by our instruments. Similarly, human mind is unseen, but we can begin to study its properties by measuring its effect on the body's properties, including the body's electromagnetic field (generated by both the brain and the heart). Members of multiple scientific disciplines, from physics to neuroscience, are beginning to formulate methods of measuring the field of consciousness so it can be studied objectively.

Something important to grasp from this discussion is that, when examining, experiencing, and maintaining your internal world, the present inability of scientific instruments to detect or describe your experience should not delude you into dismissing profound developmental experiences as "hallucination," "coincidence," or "imagination." Modern science is only just beginning to understand the intricate, invisible relationship between consciousness and the apparently external world. To connect with your inner being is to understand when to trust and how to work with the information available to your unconscious mind.

Looking to quantum physics, the currently accepted scientific description of the fundamental nature of our universe, we discover that the concept of quantum entanglement mirrors the relationship between mind, brain, consciousness, and the objective world. Chapter Four will expand the concept of entanglement with practical explanation and informative practices you can use to build your internal understanding of these exciting concepts that exist at the boundary of modern science.

In terms of spiritual teaching, understanding the field of consciousness and super-consciousness has been explored and explained through many methods, including storytelling, poems, literature, and script. Thirteenth century Persian poet and Sufi mystic Moulana Rumi skillfully explained the profound philosophy behind of the nature of consciousness, in comparison with our limited understanding of it:

The Elephant in a Dark Room (translated by Edward Henry Whinfield)[6]

> *Some Hindoos were exhibiting an elephant in a dark room, and many people collected to see it. But as the place was too dark to permit them to see the elephant, they all felt it with their hands, to gain an idea of what it was like. One felt its trunk, and declared that the beast resembled a water-pipe; another felt its ear, and said it must be a large fan; another its leg, and thought it must be a pillar; another felt its back, and declared the beast must be like a great throne. According to the part which each felt, he gave a different description of the animal.*

Chapter Three: Human Consciousness

The eye of outward sense is as the palm of a hand,

The whole of the object is not grasped in the palm.

The sea itself is one thing, the foam another;

Neglect the foam, and regard the sea with your eyes.

Waves of foam rise from the sea night and day,

You look at the foam ripples and not the mighty sea.

We, like boats, are tossed hither and thither,

We are blind though we are on the bright ocean.

Ah! you who are asleep in the boat of the body,

You see the water; behold the Water of waters!

Under the water you see there is another Water moving it,

Within the spirit is a Spirit that calls it.

Keep silence that you may hear Him speaking

Words unutterable by tongue in speech.

Keep silence, that you may hear from that Sun

Things inexpressible in books and discourses.

Insight Job

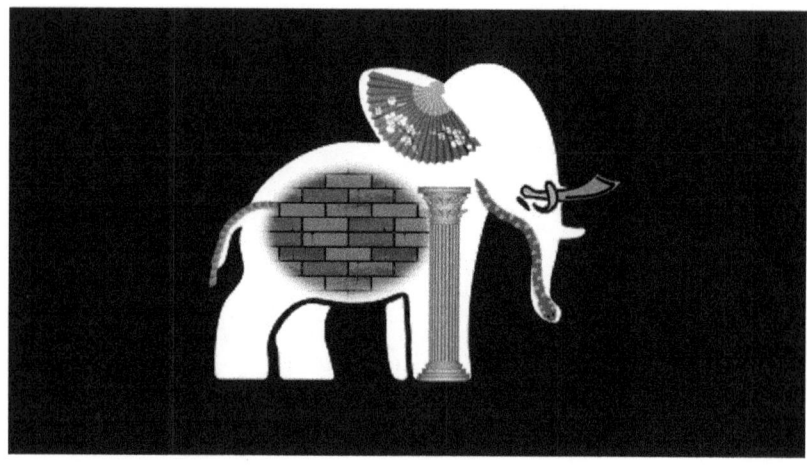

Understanding that you are indeed connected to everyone and everything around you is no longer a mystery. Once aware, you need only to acknowledge the hub of consciousness that connects one entity to another to ignite your candle of consciousness. Connecting with this realm of consciousness can renew our belief in our own potential and capacity, as well as expand our view of possibilities for our society in terms of both spirituality and science.

In spiritual terms, the "Elephant in a Dark Room" invites you first to participate in a search of the truth that resonates with you. Then, once established in that truth, you can choose to continue by either clinging only to this partial understanding of truth (i.e., preconception and prejudice) or by valuing and respecting other belief systems to let the collective understating illuminate the entire body of truth. Acceptance of the unity of all religions and spiritual practices and their mutual purpose in expanding the domain of higher realms of reality is the essential element in vanquishing dualism and making peace with oneself, communities, nations, and the human race.

Chapter Three: Human Consciousness

In technological terms, the concept of connecting to a higher realm of reality and possibilities is thoroughly analogous to a computer and its Internet connection. You, as an individual, are the super intelligent machine (analogous to a computer) that can operate at a certain capacity when left by itself. Your plans for how to use this machine to its maximum potential and even what to use it for in the first place would change substantially if you were told that it can be connected to a higher layer of information and intelligence (such as a locally connected server or globally connected Internet network). This is indeed the situation. Knowingly or unknowingly, we are all already connected to this network and influence its traffic in various ways. For the sake of everyone on the network, it is necessary that you know your multidimensional self and its capacity, connection, and relation to other forms of consciousness, whether or not you choose consciously to participate in the larger networks.

In the following weeks, you will establish (or empower previously established) pathways from the human mind and body (computer) to the flow of consciousness (Internet and servers) in the world around us. In these practices, we will be using the **human heart** as our network hardware (modem) to modulate the consciousness flow.

Now you may ask: *Why are we choosing the heart, and how are we going to practice with it?*

Beside the fact that many ancient spiritual practices and modern religions view the human heart as the sacred center of The Divine in the human body and the internal compass for life's journey, scientific evidence also exists on the importance and the power of the human heart. HeartMath Institute Director of Research Rollin McCraty writes about human heart and its abilities in the paper titled "The Energetic Heart: Bioelectromagnetic Communication Within and Between People."

Insight Job

The heart is a sensory organ and acts as a sophisticated information encoding and processing center that enables it to learn, remember, and make independent functional decisions. The heart, like the brain, generates a powerful electromagnetic field. The heart generates the largest electromagnetic field in the body. The electrical field as measured in an electrocardiogram (ECG) is about 60 times greater in amplitude than the brain waves recorded in an electroencephalogram (EEG).[7]

In another paper, "Emotional Stress, Positive Emotions, and Psychophysiological Coherence," HeartMath Institute researchers McCraty and Dana Tomasin explain the power of the energetic heart this way:

Through the use of tools and technologies that foster positive emotions and psychophysiological coherence, individuals can effectively initiate a re-patterning process, whereby habitual emotional patterns underlying stress are replaced with new, healthier patterns that establish increased emotional stability, mental acuity, and physiological efficiency as a new familiar baseline or norm.[8]

In the final chapter, you will begin to understand and activate the virtues of the heart to synchronize its communication patterns with those of the global and universal networks, growing closer to yourself, your values, and our shared humanity in the process.

End of Chapter Three

Chapter Four
HUMAN HEART

IN THE FOLLOWING WEEKS, you will explore your ability to both cultivate (generate) and accept (receive) the seven virtues of the human heart. These quests are sensitive. You should participate in these practices daily, but within your comfort zone, at your natural pace and rhythm, and away from any tension or force. Having journeyed this far into your story, you have honed your ability to direct your focus intentionally. The state of your practice may have evolved to the point at which you can consistently dedicate attention and willpower to the genuine understanding of each heart virtue throughout your daily interactions with the world around you: in any situation, with any others, and even alone with yourself.

The depth of your practice in this final chapter lies in your hands (and in your heart). You could choose to simply focus your practice on raising awareness toward the existing examples of these virtues in your day to day interactions. To expand your development, you may additionally set an intention to increase your daily generation of heart virtues, performing actions that express heart-based qualities during your daily life. If you allow this practice to guide you all the way to its natural fulfillment, you can eventually attain the experience of being wholly absorbed in each virtue, becoming a living example of the heart in action and directly embodying the supreme joy that these qualities can provide to you and those connected to you. To allow these virtues to act through you is to join yourself with the wisdom of consciousness. You are now ready to begin the practice presented in Week One.

Chapter Four: Human Heart

Week One: Virtue of Authenticity

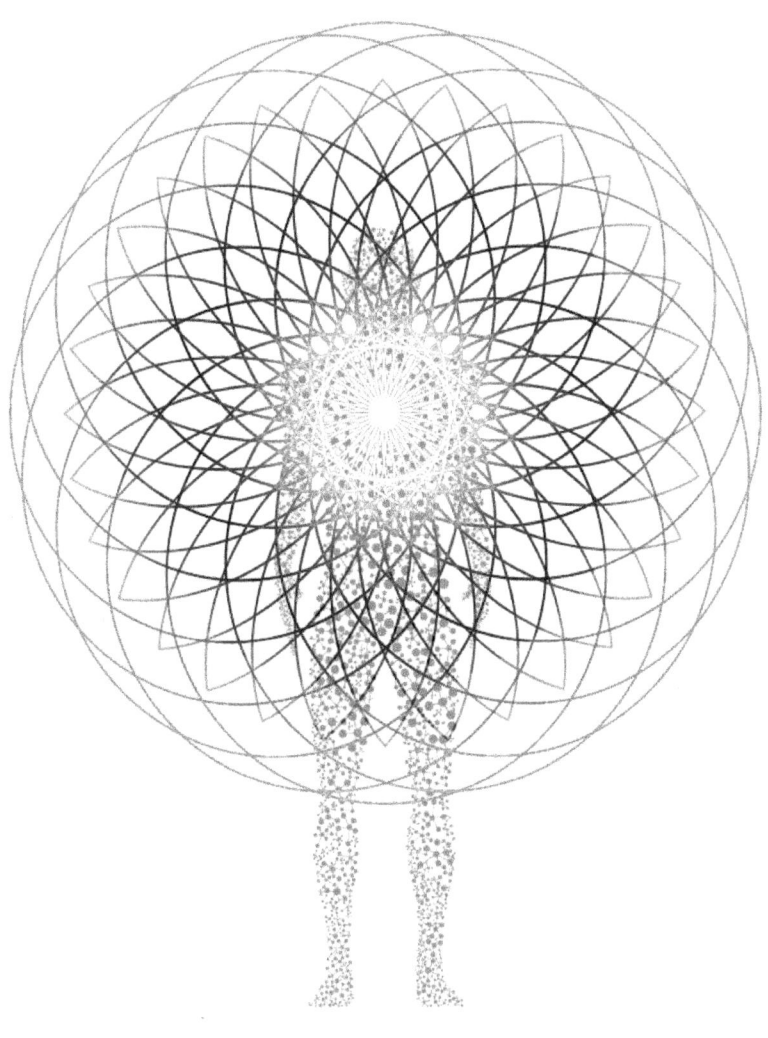

QUEST 4A
VIRTUE OF AUTHENTICITY

This week, begin your heart practice by focusing on the most important virtue in personal and professional development: Authenticity. For most, the lack of authenticity is easy to detect in others, but identifying your own authentic self and allowing that spontaneity to truly show through often presents more of a challenge.

Authenticity is the fundamental factor in building an honorable relationship with yourself and others. To be authentic is not to be faultless, but to be the genuine you.

As we saw in Chapter Two, we sometimes inadvertently identify with toxins that can inhabit various layers of our human system. As these toxins are not your true self, they can promptly dissipate when exposed to the light of your authenticity.

Chapter Four: Human Heart

Observation and Action

This week, begin by raising your awareness of the following concepts throughout the entirety of your daily experience:

- Defining your truest self
- Defining your perspective of the world
- Defining your relation with the world
- Understanding your true desires
- Understanding your true values
- Understanding your intentions

At the end of each day, set aside a window of 20 to 40 minutes to contemplate your authentic self and how much you were able to let your intentions shine through your actions. The beauty of this quest is that it will benefit you in maintaining your personal and universal moralities, because if you're *being* authentic, then your intentions, words, and action must be aligned.

Duration and Frequency

Focus on your authenticity throughout all your interactions over the course of one week.

Record your 20 to 40 minutes of reflection in your Quest Log at the end of each day.

4A

Insight Job

QUEST LOG 4A
DAY ONE

Date:

Today's reflection on the Virtue of Authenticity:

Chapter Four: Human Heart

QUEST LOG 4A
DAY TWO

Date:

Today's reflection on the Virtue of Authenticity:

Week Two: Virtue of Understanding

After spending a week exploring your authentic self, you may have noticed that, just by raising your awareness toward this virtue, you have naturally increased the chance of **being** (not *becoming*, but simply being) your true self in your own ways. If so, you are ready to move forward with Week Two to practice the next virtue. You may also spend more time on the first virtue if needed.

Advantageously, once you begin to enjoy the experience of your authentic self, you find you naturally become more **understanding** of yourself and others. You can now easily explain the underlying reasons behind your true-self actions, describe the purpose and meaning of your intentions, and provide genuine justification for all your choices. You may even start to have a clearer idea of what you need to do in the future, why, and how you are going to accomplish it within your lifetime. This level of understanding begins to affect your interaction with the world around you, including other people, nature, and other beings. It informs your perspective on all life situations including past and future events, and this is how:

Your authentic self is a combination of your physical systems (human body in three dimensions: Chapter One) with your non-physical systems (layers of the human mind as well as consciousness in the fourth dimension and above: Chapters Two and Three). Through the alignment of your intentions (purposeful thoughts), words, and actions (behaviors), you activate the heart center and allow the energy (information) of consciousness to flow from the non-physical (e.g., mental, emotional) state to the physical state, creating a new structural platform for your personal reality and experience of life. In this state, you experience the reality of your human form as a multidimensional system—a system that

Chapter Four: Human Heart

simultaneously interacts with similar systems (other humans) as well as other forms of existence (the surrounding environment, other living beings, the planet, different forms of consciousness, and more).

Considering the statement above, once you access your authentic self and become aware of its actions, you realize the effect that *you* have on other systems and see more clearly how surrounding and surrounded (internal) systems affect you, too. This realization, or level of understanding, is essential as it unlocks the next five virtues of the human heart.

This week, I encourage you to focus daily on translating your interactions with self, others, and the world around you into the concept of entanglement:

> *When two systems, of which we know the states by their respective representatives, enter into temporary physical interaction due to known forces between them, and when after a time of mutual influence the systems separate again, then they can no longer be described in the same way as before, viz. by endowing each of them with a representative of its own. I would not call that one but rather the characteristic trait of quantum mechanics, the one that enforces its entire departure from classical lines of thought. By the interaction, the two representatives [the quantum states] have become entangled.*[9]

Erwin Schrödinger, quoted above, coined the term "entanglement" to describe this extraordinary connection between quantum systems. When viewed as a concept that describes our own interaction with the universe, we can identify several different types of entanglement that we are subject to in our life experience. These can be described as follows:

Self-Entanglement

Self-Entanglement involves more than just understanding the classical co-relation between human body and mind systems. It also means your internal systems can impact each other outside the conditions of time and space, bending the laws of classical physics. Spiritualism links the self-entanglement concept to the "mind over matter" tactic often employed to overcome fears.

In scientific terms, this could be referred to as epigenetics, the field that was explained by Bruce Lipton as the "study of cellular and physiological traits or the external and environmental factors that turn the human genes on and off and, in turn, define how our cells actually read those genes."[10]

Social-Entanglement

Entanglement manifests as a somehow puzzling correlation between parties who once came into contact, and maintain their contact even miles away. This has been experimentally demonstrated with individual atoms or light beams: but how can it fit in our everyday experience of life? The closest feeling which comes into my mind is love. Think of a mother and a child, or two lovers who shared an intense emotion, and are now living at the opposite sides of the world. They feel each other, perceive the happiness or the sadness of the distant partner, and are influenced by this. Schrödinger added: 'Another way of expressing the peculiar situation is: the best possible knowledge of a whole does not necessarily include the best possible knowledge of all its parts. The lack of knowledge is due to the interaction itself.' In our metaphor, nobody of the two lovers is complete on its own. Only when taken together, they complement each other. They are

Chapter Four: Human Heart

non-separable halves of the same entangled entity. No proper and complete understanding, on both physical and psychological grounds, is available for this phenomenon. But the language of art, probably, can make it clearer: entanglement is admirably depicted by Pamela Ott, who has almost zero knowledge of quantum mechanics (I asked her!) and paints 'from her subconscious'. The waveness of the lines, the choice of complimentary colors, the faded entwining of bodies and souls is what in my opinion most closely resembles a true image of entanglement, and of loving passion.

Professor Gerardo Adesso[11]

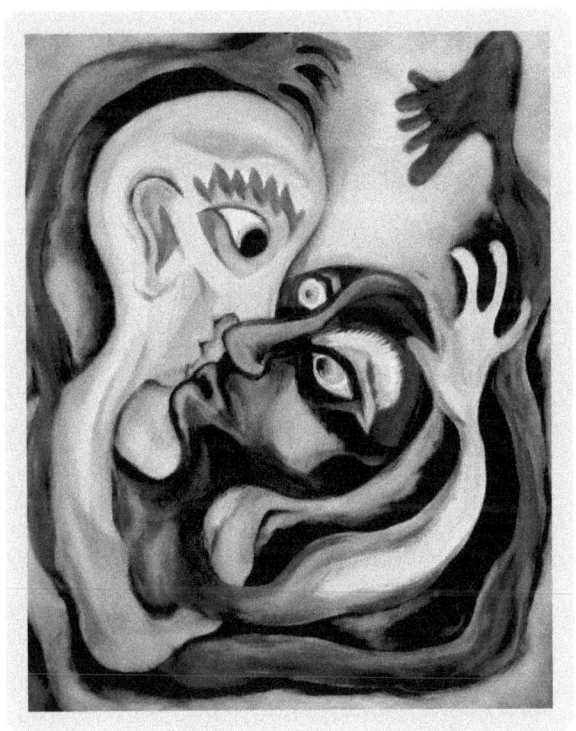

Surroundings-Entanglement

While Self-Entanglement and Social-Entanglement always affect us, the practice of Surroundings-Entanglement is more of a voluntary interpersonal communication with entities around you. To feel this level of entanglement changes our environmental awareness and the way we interact with our surroundings. Martin Buber, the twentieth-century philosopher best known for his book Ich und Du (I and Thou),[12] explains the two types interaction that a human can have with his or her surroundings in terms of I-It and I-Thou dialogues. Buber's attempt to identify the bidirectional dialogue between humans and their surroundings was an open invitation to practice Surroundings-Entanglement—an invitation to shift the I-It towards the I-Thou:

> I-It: the attitude of objective separation from the "I" (human) towards an "It" (surroundings: other humans, animals, environment, etc.)

> I-Thou: The attitude of subjective non-separation from the "I" towards "Thou" (presence of the reflection of Thou in all things)

The voluntary acknowledgment of the intertwined relationship between you and your surroundings allows you to see how your intentions and actions can make a difference in our environment and how our environment's intentions and actions can make a difference in you.

Chapter Four: Human Heart

Situation-Entanglement

The correlation of situation entanglement could be understood through posing the famous question: *Do men make history or does history make men?*

When trying to answer the question of which variable is dependent on the other, you may consider many examples in our history, and find a strange co-relation between the variables, yet no definite answer. Therefore, when the question of the importance of our history arises (beyond an attempt to avoid repeating mistakes), Situation-Entanglement demonstrates its value in making more clear our understanding of how the past relates (or doesn't relate) to our current state of being or potential, future events. Holding onto ideas about—or making decisions based on—a picture of the past that does not include an understanding of the situation that each involved party was subject to at the time can lead to confusion or unnecessarily held resentment.

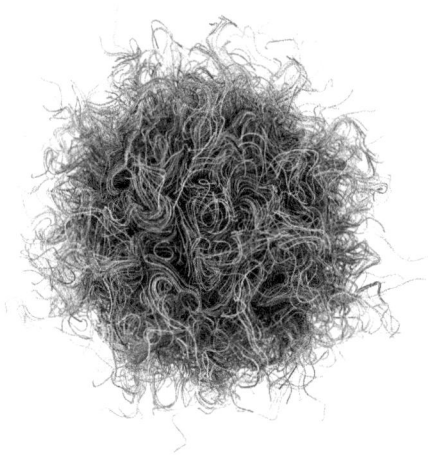

Insight Job

Superconscious-Entanglement:

The last form of entanglement we will review is perhaps the deepest form: Superconscious-Entanglement. A good introduction to Superconscious-Entanglement is a thought experiment related to the ancient belief of pantheism, which views that God consists only of everything in the (multidimensional) universe and that there can be no God distinct from the universe itself (and the laws of physics therein). To take from this view that each thing in this reality of the universe is identical to the super-consciousness of God (the entire universe) is an obvious logical and spiritual fallacy. However, in the domain of spiritual thought, it is seen as true that the universe and all existence (which, it is apparent, contains our consciousness) had to be created by, created out of, stem from, or reflect a higher level of conscious existence, as we are ourselves conscious.

For example, the human mind is the source of all technological inventions. Therefore, all technological inventions are the reflections of the human mind, but only to the extent of their limitations. Clearly, you cannot fully comprehend the human mind through any, or even every, invention; however, you can confirm that in all human inventions you can find the presence of the human mind. Similarly, it is also must be true that all things manifested (consciously created) in the universe are the reflections of the conscious creator (The Divine, God, higher dimensional physics) only to their own extent. Likewise, in the spiritual belief of pantheism, to consider all forms of consciousness as identical to the super-consciousness of The Divine is as invalid as to believe you can fully comprehend all layers of the human mind through a single invention.

In the same example, depending on the level of intelligence or complexity of the invention, the correlation between the inventor and the invention changes. For instance, a laptop computer is a much deeper representation

Chapter Four: Human Heart

of the human mind than a digital watch. But because they were both created (*informed*) by the human mind, we can research them to gain *infor*mation about the mind of their creator. Throughout scientific history, this co-relation between creator and creation has allowed the pantheists and the super-consciousness of The Divine to bidirectionally communicate information through the universe. Superconscious-Entanglement explains this level of communication. Throughout the history of spiritual, scientific, and artistic discovery, we can see clearly the world-altering and mind-expanding effects of Superconscious-Entanglement in the works of many pantheists such as Albert Einstein, Beethoven, Nikola Tesla, Carl Jung, Alan Watts, Leo Tolstoy, and many more.

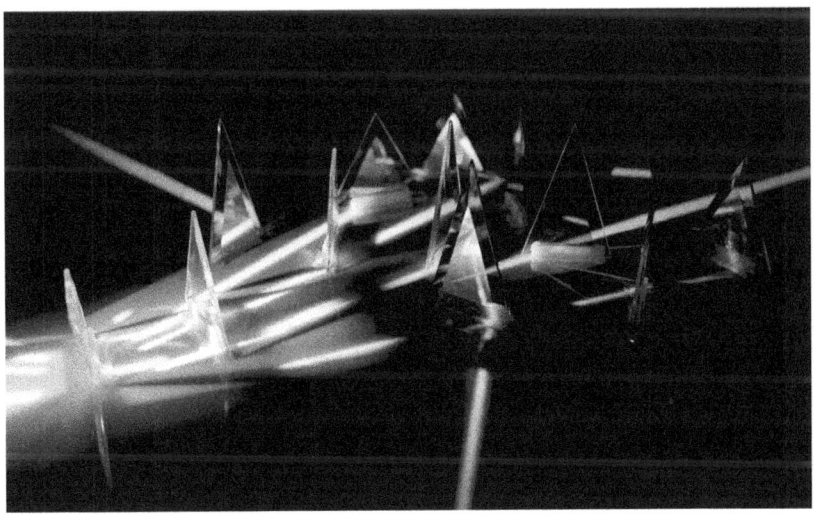

QUEST 4B
VIRTUE OF UNDERSTANDING

Observation and Action

This week, dedicate attention, throughout the entirety of your daily experience, to the understanding of how the concepts presented in this chapter are influencing your life. Review the following concepts each morning:

Self-Entanglement

Social-Entanglement

Surroundings-Entanglement

Situation-Entanglement

Superconscious-Entanglement

At the end of each day, set aside an open window of 20 to 40 minutes to translate your day's interactions with self, others, and the world around you into these concepts of entanglement.

Chapter Four: Human Heart

Duration and Frequency

Focus on the various forms of entanglement throughout all your interactions over the course of one week.

Record your 20 to 40 minutes of reflection in your Quest Log at the end of each day.

4B

Insight Job

QUEST LOG 4B
DAY ONE

Date:
Today's reflection on entanglement:

Chapter Four: Human Heart

QUEST LOG 4B
DAY ONE

Date:

Today's reflection on entanglement:

Week Three: Virtue of Forgiveness

Once your authentic-self gains enough awareness to align your intentions, words, and actions, you begin to understand the relationship between you and others through the principles of entanglement. As you practice (*intend to connect to*) the Virtue of Understanding and it becomes integrated (*downloaded*) into your human system, it will naturally reveal its outward expression (*activate its program*): **forgiveness**.

The Virtue of Forgiveness is the key to liberation from the judgment of the past and the inevitable changes of the present and future. Understanding the connection between your mind and body, yourself and others, your surroundings and your life situations, and how all of this is linked to super-consciousness brings you to the point of **non-judgment**. This is because, while you may not be fully aware of other systems intentions, actions, and behaviors, you recognize that, like yourself, their expressions and interactions are also influenced by many other entangled factors (of which neither you nor they are fully aware). Consequently, you could not possibly judge what appears to be their objective (independent) behavior, as it has been initiated wholly or partially by subjective (dependent) factors through entanglement principles. When the authority of judgment is taken away from you by the light of your own awareness, you begin to **accept** what is. You begin to accept yourself, others, life circumstances, and the higher power through your own understanding. You let go of whatever cannot be understood and/or accepted through this process. This letting-go in good faith is the Virtue of Forgiveness. The beauty of this virtue is that you can practice it from the smallest to the most complex circumstances beyond the condition of time or space. This means you can travel through your heart and mind to a different time or space to initiate forgiveness. This is one of the first multidimensional practices in this book.

Chapter Four: Human Heart

A deep human being feels pain and allows oneself to suffer because that's part of the human experience. Without acknowledging that you've been wounded and you've lost something, you don't gain the benefit of the experience—of acknowledging that you've been hurt and mistreated, but also of healing. And so there is a power that comes from the experience. But a deep human being also lets go of their suffering—he or she doesn't maintain it forever, doesn't create his or her personality around it, doesn't use it as a weapon. You don't cling to the negative part of the experience so that you can have something to hold accountable for your failures.

Fred Luskin, Ph.D.[13]

QUEST 4C
VIRTUE OF FORGIVENESS

Observation and Action

This week, focus your awareness and action toward forgiveness throughout the entirety of your daily experience. Start by considering minor subjects and slowly approach more sensitive matters once you feel prepared. Fortunately, it is very easy to find opportunities to forgive others, your surroundings, and, most importantly, yourself in daily life. If focusing more deeply on this practice, you may be surprised to find how many small events in your day can serve as objects of your forgiveness, saving you from generating micro-negativity that can accumulate to weigh you down. You can forgive the mosquito for biting you, the sidewalk for tripping you, the taxi driver for cutting you off, your back for aching, your mind for generating unwelcome thoughts, and much more. In addition, you can reinforce your practice by focusing on the feeling of lightness or relief that each act of forgiveness conveys.

At the end of each day, spend your 20 to 40 minutes of daily contemplation either to continue practicing forgiveness or to consider and record your acts of forgiveness that occurred throughout the day and how they made you feel (and whether you feel they are, indeed, completely forgiven).

You can also include contemplation and action based on the following instruction, provided by Fred Luskin, Ph.D., director of

Chapter Four: Human Heart

the Stanford University Forgiveness Project and the author of *Forgive for Good: A Proven Prescription for Health and Happiness.*

The first step is to fully acknowledge the harm done, whether by you or somebody else, and to own the fact that you've lost something—that you didn't get something you wanted, and it hurts. In a therapeutic context, that could be painful work. Sometimes it takes therapeutic work before somebody's ready to forgive because they've suppressed a bad experience or been in denial about it, and it may take an effort to get them to acknowledge the harm or its consequences.

The second step of the grief process is to experience the feelings normally associated with the negative experience. It's not enough just to have someone say, "Hey, I was beaten for 12 years and I want to get over it" if they've never been miserable about their suffering. They're going to have to be miserable before they let it go. I've never met anyone who suffered real loss and didn't suffer at some level. You experience a range of emotions—you're sad, you're scared. But when you forgive, you understand that there are other options besides continued suffering. You're not letting go of the event—that's immutable. But you can transform the emotional response to it.

The third and final step is that what you're grieving can't be a secret. I try not to let people forgive stuff that they haven't shared with others because there's such good research on resilience showing that people who go through harmful experiences and don't tell anybody have much worse consequences than people who do tell others. The human connection is central to healing.[13]

Remember that by holding back forgiveness and maintaining a negative response to the memory of a situation you affect your own well-being (often more than you are affecting the would-be object of your forgiveness). It has been found that forgiveness can lower blood pressure and heart rate as well as reducing levels of depression, anxiety, and anger. People who tend to forgive generally have more and better relationships with others, feel happier and more hopeful, and score higher on just about every measure of psychological well-being.

Duration and Frequency

Focus on forgiveness throughout all your interactions over the course of one week.

Record your 20 to 40 minutes of reflection in your Quest Log at the end of each day.

4C

Insight Job

QUEST LOG 4C
DAY ONE

Date:

Today's reflection on the Virtue of Forgiveness:

Chapter Four: Human Heart

QUEST LOG 4C
DAY TWO

Date:

Today's reflection on the Virtue of Forgiveness:

Week Four: Virtue of Allowance

As you begin to experience the joys of truthfulness, understanding, and forgiveness, you find yourself in the state of calmness and **tranquility**. This state of mind encourages you to **trust** your true, authentic self (including your intentions and actions) more than ever before. Through this **integrity**, you also form a stronger bond of trust and **honor** with everything and everyone around you. With this trust, you learn that once you act in terms of being authentic to yourself and others and participate in understanding and forgiveness, you have done your part. Thereby, whether you believe in a higher power in religious terms or have **faith** in the **goodness** of *your own actions* (i.e., karma), you will be content with the outcome of your interactions. The state of inner belief and **contentment** is the outward expression of the Virtue of **Allowance**. Allowance is to admit that you are not the only creator or beneficiary of your life experience and reality, then to acknowledge that other systems in this time and space also participate in shaping your experience and our reality. Through the art of allowance, you, as an individual system, join other individual systems to co-create a collective experience and co-shape a semi-permanent or temporary frame of reality. The practice of allowance generates other possibilities in terms of how you perceive the world around you. In other words, through allowance you can elevate your perception beyond the condition of time and space (described by some as "the law of attraction").

Consider that sometimes in life you do not have the authority to change the circumstances. You may then have to trust in yourself and/or a higher power and surrender. The truth is that if we expand the timescale of our view on a situation, we often find ourselves looking back after some

Chapter Four: Human Heart

time to realize what appeared to be troublesome was, in fact, necessary for our own growth or to unlock a timeline of later experience that was dependent on the seemingly negative event occurring exactly as it did.

The trouble is in the mind, for the body is only the house for the mind to dwell in, and we put a value on it according to its worth. Therefore if your mind has been deceived by some invisible enemy into a belief, you have put it into the form of a disease, with or without your knowledge. By my theory or truth, I come in contact with your enemy and restore you to your health and happiness. This I do partly mentally and partly by talking till I correct the wrong impressions and establish the Truth, and the Truth is the cure.

From *The Quimby Manuscripts* by Phineas Parkhurst Quimby[14]

QUEST 4D
VIRTUE OF ALLOWANCE

Observation and Action

This week, engage your mind and heart in the practice of allowance. Each day, give yourself 20 to 40 minutes to sit in meditation with the previous events of your life in mind. Think of all the seemingly negative events that led to positive endings. Contemplate the multitude of entangled circumstances behind a major personal development. Consider a time you narrowly escaped trauma, then recognize the minor inconveniences that diverted your path from danger into safety. Imagine the learning opportunities that stemmed from the traumatic events that did unfold in your life.

Using the same technique, practice allowance throughout your day to generate heart-based trust and faith towards your current life situations that you do not have the power to control.

Duration and Frequency

Focus on allowance throughout all your interactions over the course of one week.

Record your 20 to 40 minutes of reflection in your Quest Log at the end of each day.

QUEST LOG 4D
DAY ONE

Date:

Today's reflection on the Virtue of Allowance:

Chapter Four: Human Heart

QUEST LOG **4D**
DAY TWO

Date:

Today's reflection on the Virtue of Allowance:

Week Five: Virtue of Balance

After working with the Virtue of Allowance, practitioners may find themselves in an inevitable mental trap. The fine line between taking responsibility for your intentions and actions (entanglement principles of your doing affecting your system and others) and accepting the dark side of reality that you cannot control everything that happens to you (Virtue of Allowance) could cause an illusion of duality.

To believe that your voluntary thoughts and behaviors can fully control and shape your life experience is to consider your mind the only creator of this reality. In this case, your free will is the only one to praise or blame for everything that happens in your entire life. Do you think your authentic self could pridefully take credit for every good thing that happened to you while guiltily faulting yourself for every single matter that ever went wrong?

On the other hand, could you convince yourself that your entire life experience has been written into the tomes of destiny and you have no choice but to allow it to be? In that case, nothing (remarkably positive or awfully negative) that you do or have ever done towards yourself or others matters due to the nature of absolute determinism. In this case, do you find yourself treated fairly or victimized?

This extreme polarity between absolute **free will** (everything that you do matters) and absolute **determinism** (nothing that you do matters) brings us to a point of awareness: the need for **balance**.

The ancient Virtue of Balance is one of the most fundamental principles of both personal and universal moralities.

Chapter Four: Human Heart

At the very roots of Chinese thinking and feeling there lies the principle of polarity, which is not to be confused with the ideas of opposition or conflict. In the metaphors of other cultures, light is at war with darkness, life with death, good with evil, and the positive with the negative, and thus an idealism to cultivate the former and be rid of the latter flourishes throughout much of the world. To the traditional way of Chinese thinking this is as incomprehensible as an electric current without both positive and negative poles, for polarity is the principle that plus and minus, north and south, are different aspects of one and the same system, and that the disappearance of either one of them would be the disappearance of the system. In Chinese the two poles of cosmic energy are yang (positive) and yin (negative), associated with the masculine and the feminine, the firm and the yielding, the strong and the weak, the light and the dark, the rising and the falling, heaven and earth, and they are even recognized in such everyday matters as cooking as the spicy and the bland. Thus the art of life is not seen as holding to yang and banishing yin, but as keeping the two in balance, because there cannot be one without the other. The key to the relationship between yang and yin is called hsiang sheng, mutual arising or inseparability. As Lao-tzu puts it:

Insight Job

When everyone knows beauty as beautiful,

there is already ugliness;

When everyone knows good as goodness,

there is already evil.

"To be" and "not to be" arise mutually;

Difficult and easy are mutually realized;

Long and short are mutually contrasted;

High and low are mutually posited;

Before and after are in mutual sequence.

They are thus like the different, but inseparable, sides of a coin, the poles of a magnet, or pulse and interval in any vibration. There is never the ultimate possibility that either one will win over the other, for they are more like lovers wrestling than enemies fighting.

It is difficult in our logic to see that being and non-being are mutually generative and mutually supportive, for it is the great and imaginary terror of Western man that nothingness will be the permanent universe. We do not easily grasp the point that the void is creative, and that being comes from non-being as sound from silence and light from space. Thus the yin-yang principle is that the somethings and the nothings, the ons and the offs, the solids and the spaces, as well as the wakings and the sleepings and the alternations of existing and not existing, are mutually necessary.

Alan Watts on Taoism[15]

Chapter Four: Human Heart

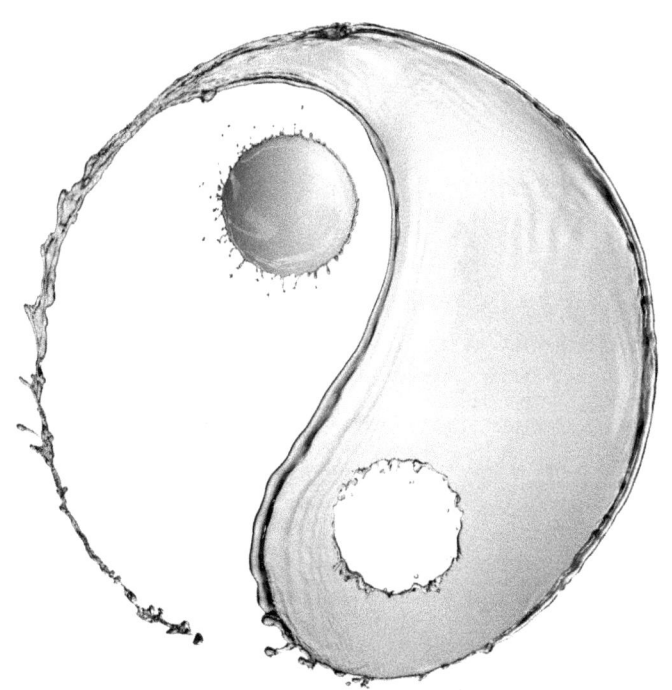

QUEST 4E
VIRTUE OF BALANCE

Observation and Action

This week, dedicate your daily practice of 20 to 40 minutes to contemplate balance in your life. Consider the two sides of reality: co-creation of your life experience through partial free will and partial determinism. The concept of balance pervades the entire life experience. Where could you apply the precious Virtue of Balance in your personal life? What parts of your life feel unbalanced, and how could you nudge them back toward the center or allow them to center naturally? Where do you see that your voluntary actions (free will) could change the circumstance, and where can you accept the nature of determinism and surrender to the unchangeable?

Duration and Frequency

Focus on balance throughout all your activities over the course of one week.

Record your 20 to 40 minutes of contemplation in your Quest Log at the end of each day.

4E

Chapter Four: Human Heart

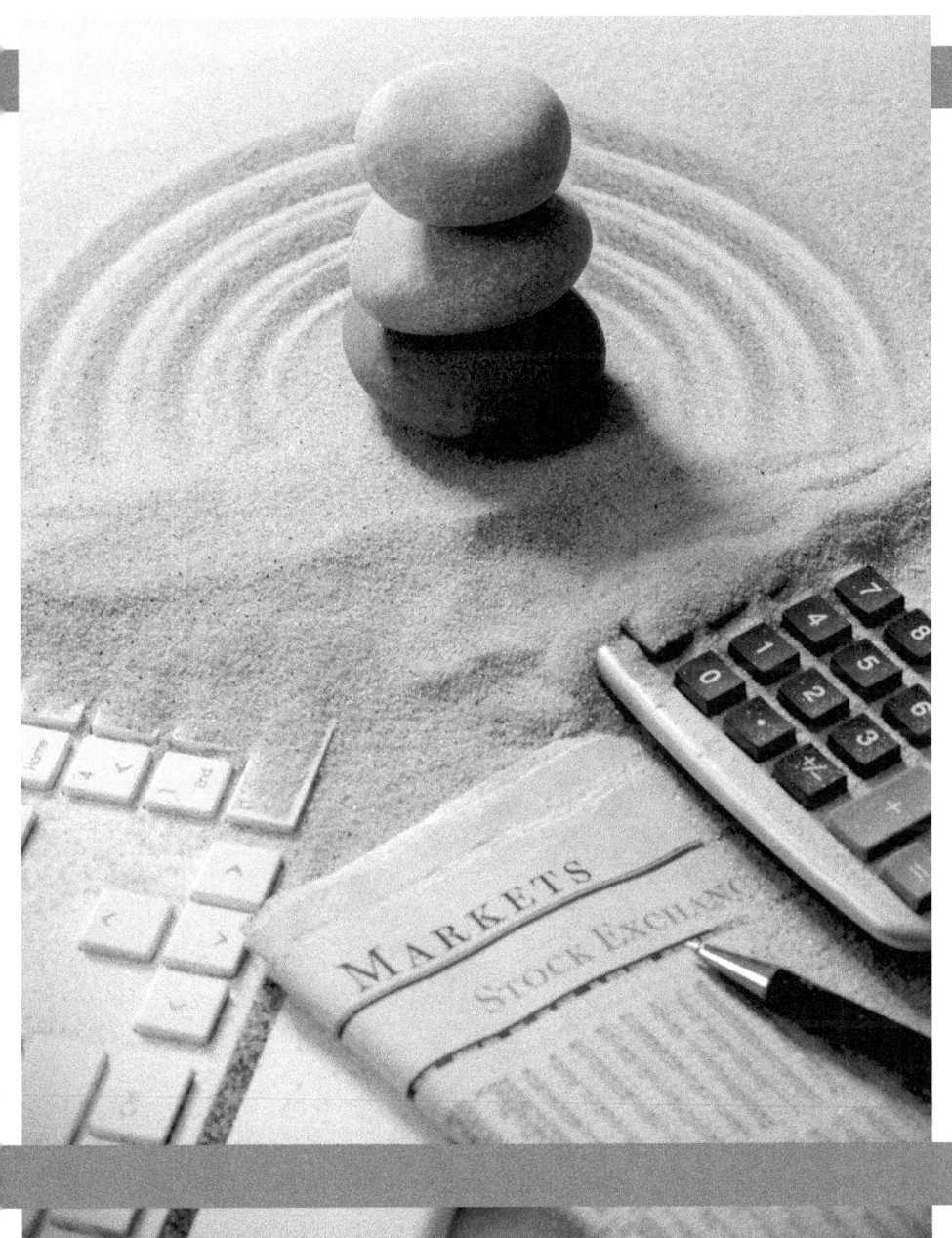

Insight Job

QUEST LOG 4E
DAY ONE

Date:

Today's contemplation on the Virtue of Balance:

Chapter Four: Human Heart

QUEST LOG 4E
DAY TWO

Date:

Today's contemplation on the Virtue of Balance:

Week Six: Virtue of Unity

"We are here to awaken from the illusion of our separateness."

Thich Nhat Hanh[16]

The Virtue of Balance prepares the conditions of the human mind and heart to work respectfully with the opposite poles of reality and everything in between. Experiencing this state of **respect** allows you to recognize that our participation in the co-creation of a unified realm of reality is manifested in diversity. This means everything and everyone that is part of this reality which shapes your life experience (perception) is also involved in its manifestation in various ways. Some might contribute toward what appears to be negative, some may enhance what appears to be positive.

"The yin-yang principle is not, therefore, what we would ordinarily call a dualism, but rather an explicit duality expressing an implicit unity."

Alan Watts[15]

Chapter Four: Human Heart

The Virtue of **Unity** allows you to **transcend** your ordinary need of belongingness to assume the extraordinary experience of living in **harmony** with all. In this practice of unity, you learn to connect with other systems and appreciate their state of existence as well. Through the Virtue of Unity, you free yourself from the illusion of separation.

"Our separation from each other is an optical illusion."

Albert Einstein[17]

Einstein called entanglement "spooky action at a distance," because the contemporary understanding was of local actions. It was spooky to think distant objects could have a direct influence on one another, because an object was seen as only being directly influenced by its immediate surroundings. The concept of entanglement in quantum theories was later supported by Nonlocality Theory of John Bell (Bell's Theorem), which suggested that objects could influence one another from distance and communicate on a non-local level according to entanglement principles.

When the fabric of reality is examined very closely, nothing resembling clockworks can be found. Instead, the reality is woven from strange, "holistic" threads that aren't located precisely in space or time. Tug on a dangling loose end from this fabric of reality, and the whole cloth twitches, instantly, throughout all space and time. Science is at the very earliest stages of understanding entanglement, and much is yet to learn. But what we've seen so far provides a new way of thinking about psi [psychic phenomena]. No longer are psi experiences regarded as rare human talents, divine gifts, or "powers" that magically transcend ordinary physical boundaries.

Insight Job

Instead, psi becomes an unavoidable consequence of living in an interconnected, entangled physical reality. Psi is reframed from a bizarre anomaly that doesn't fit into the normal world—and hence labeled paranormal—into a natural phenomenon of physics.

From *Entangled Minds: Extrasensory Experiences in a Quantum Reality* by Dean Radin[18]

In many ancient spiritual practices, such as Buddhism and Sufism, practitioners are encouraged to independently investigate their reality and true-self. From the investigation of truth, ego (in Buddhism) and Nafs (in Sufism) are known to be the source of sorrow and all suffering of humankind if left in the absence of self-awareness and self-control. Most modern religions describe the ego as an instrument or a tool to transcend the human experience from the temporary illusion of separation and ignorance to the permanent reality of oneness.

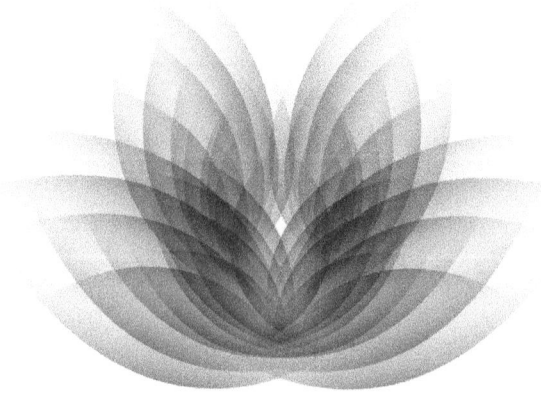

Chapter Four: Human Heart

What is non-self, Anatta? It means impermanence. If things are impermanent, they don't remain the same things forever. You of this moment are no longer you of a minute ago. There is no permanent entity within us, there is only a stream of being. There is always a lot of input and output. The input and the output happen in every second, and we should learn how to look at life as streams of being, and not as separate entities. For instance, looking into a flower, you can see that the flower is made of many elements that we can call non-flower elements. When you touch the flower, you touch the cloud. You cannot remove the cloud from the flower, because if you could remove the cloud from the flower, the flower would collapse right away. You don't have to be a poet in order to see a cloud floating in the flower, but you know very well that without the clouds there would be no rain and no water for the flower to grow. So cloud is part of the flower, and if you send the element cloud back to the sky, there will be no flower. Cloud is a non-flower element. And the sunshine...you can touch the sunshine here. If you send back the element sunshine, the flower will vanish. And sunshine is another non-flower element. And earth, and gardener... if you continue, you will see a multitude of non-flower elements in the flower. In fact, a flower is made only with non-flower elements. It does not have a separate self.

So a flower is described as empty. But I like to say it differently. A flower is empty only of a separate self, but a flower is full of everything else. The whole cosmos can be seen, can be identified, and can be touched, in one flower. So to say that the flower is empty of a separate self also means that the flower is full of the cosmos. It's the same thing. So you are of the same nature as a flower: you are empty of a separate self, but you are full of the cosmos. You are as wonderful as the cosmos, you are a manifestation of the cosmos.

From *The Island of Self* by Thich Nhat Hanh[16]

Looking back at our previous chapters and activities clarifies the theme of unity:

In Chapter One: You dedicated time and energy to comprehend your physical body systems to improve your health because you belong to them and they belong to you.

In Chapter Two: You explored the layers of human mind and re-connected to your conscious, subconscious, and unconscious mind to obtain mental clarity and a cohesive state of mind. You gathered your mind and thoughts, because they contribute to the platform of the structure of this reality and the experience of life. You belong to your worldview and your perception belongs to you.

In Chapter Three: You became aware of the power of your heart and its important relation to human body and mind. You recognized the ability of the human heart to cultivate (generate) and accept (receive) the consciousness flow (super-consciousness) through your intention and actions. You belong to your heart, and your heart being in the right place belongs to you.

In Chapter Four: You are in the process of identifying the human heart virtues, reuniting your mind, body, and heart (spirit, soul) to elevate your perception of the relation between you and other systems (mankind, society, other living beings, environment, and the whole universe). The practice of the human heart virtues illuminates the connection pathways between you and everything else. You belong to this realm of reality and this reality belongs to you.

Chapter Four: Human Heart

QUEST 4F
VIRTUE OF UNITY

Observation and Action

This week, dedicate your daily practice to using your conscious self and ego as an instrument to expand your sensitivity to the Virtue of Unity.

During this quest, try to differentiate the sources of your actions by investigating the actual motive of your intentions. First, make a list of your egocentric intentions and actions versus altruistic. Then contemplate how you could create a balance between the two lists through comprehending the Virtue of Unity.

Duration and Frequency

Focus on the Virtue of Unity throughout all your activities over the course of one week.

Record your 20 to 40 minutes of contemplation in your Quest Log at the end of each day.

4F

Insight Job

QUEST LOG 4F
DAY ONE

Date:

Today's list of intentions: (labeled as egocentric or altruistic)

How to create balance:

Further contemplation on the Virtue of Unity:

Chapter Four: Human Heart

QUEST LOG 4F
DAY TWO

Date:

Today's list of intentions: (labeled as egocentric or altruistic)

How to create balance:

Further contemplation on the Virtue of Unity:

Week Seven: Virtue of Compassion

Having consciously focused on the Virtue of Unity, you begin to notice the activation of your heart as you generate a sense of care for others. You notice your mind and your heart are both more sensitive to receiving information about other systems and their physical, mental, and emotional state of being. The more deeply you understand a feeling or experience within yourself, the more clearly you can see the same experience in others. You **naturally** begin to expand your frame of reality and experience the impression of unity in the form of **co-existence**. Living in harmony and peace with other forms of existence (humankind, nations, religions, other species, the environment, and the cosmos) develops a sense of responsibility and courage (**valor**) to maintain a safe environment of growth for all. With this duty also comes the **wisdom** of sympathetic consciousness for others: the Virtue of **Compassion**.

The English word *compassion* comes from Old French derived from the ecclesiastical Latin *compati* which means "to suffer with." Compassion is one of the fundamental teachings and practice concepts of all the major religions in the world. The depth of compassion depends on the depth of your understanding and practice of human heart virtues, and it can be mainly classified under two major structures:

Compassion created through direct attachment and the principle of locality

This state of compassion is the state of conditional love, which allows you to generate compassion towards those with whom you are directly involved. Your attachment to those systems determines the depth of your compassion towards them. This is also the level of conditional love and valor which is based on the level of their direct influence in your life and immediate surroundings.

Chapter Four: Human Heart

Compassion created through indirect connections and entanglement principles

This state of compassion is the state of unconditional love, which allows you to cultivate compassion toward those with whom you are indirectly involved. Your mere awareness of those systems engenders a depth of compassion toward them. Therefore, once you become aware of their existence, your heart begins to generate unconditional love towards them, regardless of your direct involvement with them.

From my own limited experience, I have found that the greatest degree of inner tranquility comes from the development of love and compassion. The more we care for the happiness of others, the greater our own sense of well-being becomes. Cultivating a close, warm-hearted feeling for others automatically puts the mind at ease. This helps remove whatever fears or insecurities we may have and gives us the strength to cope with any obstacles we encounter. It is the ultimate source of success in life. As long as we live in this world we are bound to encounter problems. If, at such times, we lose hope and become discouraged, we diminish our ability to face difficulties. If, on the other hand, we remember that it is not just ourselves but everyone who has to undergo suffering, this more realistic perspective will increase our determination and capacity to overcome troubles. Indeed, with this attitude, each new obstacle can be seen as yet another valuable opportunity to improve our mind! Thus we can strive gradually to become more compassionate, that is we can develop both genuine sympathy for others' suffering and the will to help remove their pain. As a result, our own serenity and inner strength will increase.

Dalai Lama[19]

QUEST 4G
VIRTUE OF COMPASSION

Action

This week, you are encouraged to explore the Virtue of Compassion in your own way. Begin with your own attachments, then slowly expand your sense of compassion toward other systems of which you are aware. At this point, with the authority of all seven virtues, you could easily go back to review your work with any previous quests to see how your Tree of Life has grown.

"Be the change that you wish to see in the world."

Mahatma Gandhi

"I am the change I wish to see in the world."

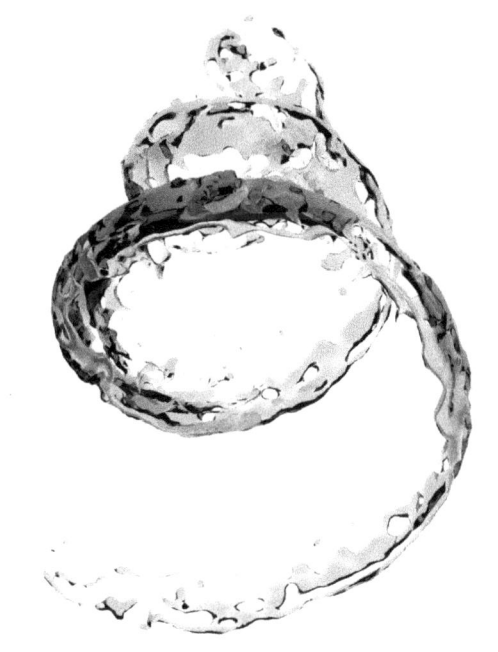

References

1. Alpert, Ram Dass Richard. "Be Here Now." By Ram Dass, 12 Oct.1-22. 1979. Print

2. James Strohl. "Multidimensional Spiritual Psychology." Founder of Multidimensional Spiritual Psychology, 26 Feb. 2016, web:http://jamesstrohl.com/multidimensional-spiritual-psychology/.

3. Weil, Andrew. "Breathing Exercise: Three to Try | 4-7-8 Breath | Andrew Weil, M.D.", 12 Dec. 2017, web:www.drweil.com/health-wellness/body-mind-spirit/stress-anxiety/breathing-three-exercises/.

4. Lipton, Bruce. "Subconscious vs Conscious." 31 Mar. 2016,web:www.brucelipton.com/blog/subconscious-vs-conscious/.

5. Lipton, Bruce. "Is There a Way to Change Subconscious Patterns?" 24 Apr. 2015, web:www.brucelipton.com/blog/there-way-change-subconscious-patterns/.

6. Jalāl al-Dīn Rūmī, Maulana.Masnavi i Man'avi, the spiritual couplets of Maulána Jalálu-d'-Dín Muhammad i Rúmí.Translated and abridged by E.H. Whinfield.London, Trubner, 1887. Print

7. McCraty, Rollin. "The Energetic Heart: Bioelectromagnetic Communication Within and Between People." HeartMath Institute. 2004,web:www.heartmath.org/research/research-library/energetics/energetic-heart-bioelectromagnetic-communication-within-and-between-people/.

8. McCraty, Rollin, and Dana Tomasino. "Emotional Stress, Positive Emotions, and Psychophysiological Coherence." HeartMath Institute. 2006,web:www.heartmath.org/research/research-library/basic/emotional-stress-positive-emotions-and-psychophysiological-coherence/.

9. Schrodinger, E.Discussion of probability relations between separated systems. Proceedings of the Cambridge Philosophical Society, 555-563. 1935. Print

10. Lipton, Bruce H.The Biology of Belief: Unleashing the Power of Consciousness, Matter & Miracles. Hay House, Inc.2016. Print

11. Adesso, Gerardo. The Social Aspects of Quantum Entanglement. 2007,web:https://arxiv.org/ftp/arxiv/papers/0706/0706.0286.pdf/.

12. 12. Buber, Martin, and Ronald Gregor. Smith. I And Thou. Bloomsbury, 2013. Print

13. Luskin, Fred. "What Is Forgiveness?" Greater Good, 19 Aug. 2010,web:https://greatergood.berkeley.edu/article/item/fred_luskin_explains_how_to_forgive/.

14. Quimby, P. P., and Horatio W. Dresser. Christ or Science: Chapter IV, the Quimby Manuscripts. Builder Press, 194. 2014. Print

15. Watts, Alan. "The Taoist View of the Universe." [1967?], Sausalito, California, Lecture.

16. Hanh, Thich Nhat. "Tag: Island of Self." Thich Nhat Hanh Dharma Talks, 30 Mar. 2014,web:https://tnhaudio.org/tag/island-of-self/.

17. Einstein, Albert." Quote by Albert Einstein: "Our Separation from Each Other Is an Optical Il...",web:www.goodreads.com/quotes/169344-our-separation-from-each-other-is-an-optical-illusion/.

18. Radin, Dean I. Entangled Minds: Extrasensory Experiences in a Quantum Reality. Paraview Pocket Books, 3.2006. Print

19. Dalai Lama. "Compassion and the Individual." The 14th Dalai Lama.2016,web:https://www.dalailama.com/messages/compassion-and-human-values/compassion/.

Resources

Buber Martín, and Shmuel Noah Eisenstadt. On Intersubjectivity and Cultural Creativity. University of Chicago Press, 1992. Print

Chalmers, David John. The Conscious Mind: in Search of a Fundamental Theory. Oxford University Press, 2007. Print

Chopra, Deepak, and Rudolph E Tanzi. The Healing Self. Harmony Books, 2018. Print

Coello, Paulo. The Alchemist. Chivers, 2003. Print

Iyengar, B. K. S. The Light on Yoga: Yoga Dipika. HarperCollins Publishers India, 1979. Print

Maehle, Gregor. Ashtanga Yoga: Practice and Philosophy: a Comprehensive Description of the Primary Series of Ashtanga Yoga, Following the Traditional Vinyasa Count, and an Authentic Explanation of the Yoga Sutra of Patanjali Patanjali. New World Library, 2008. Print

McTaggart, Lynne. The Field: the Quest for the Secret Force of the Universe. Harper, 2008. Print

Seligman, M. E. (2004). Authentic happiness: using the new positive psychology to realize your potential for lasting fulfillment. New York: Free Press. Print

Sell, Christina. My Body Is a Temple: Yoga as a Path to Wholeness. Hohm Press, 2011. Print

Suzuki, Shunryu, et al. Zen Mind, Beginner's Mind. Shambhala, 2011. Print

Willett, Walter. Eat, Drink, and be Healthy: the Harvard Medical School Guide to Healthy Eating. Free Press, 2017. Print

Zinn, J. (1991). Full catastrophe living: using the wisdom of your body and mind to face stress, pain, and illness. New York, N.Y.: Pub. By Dell Pub., a division of Bantam Doubleday Dell Pub. Group. Print

About the Author

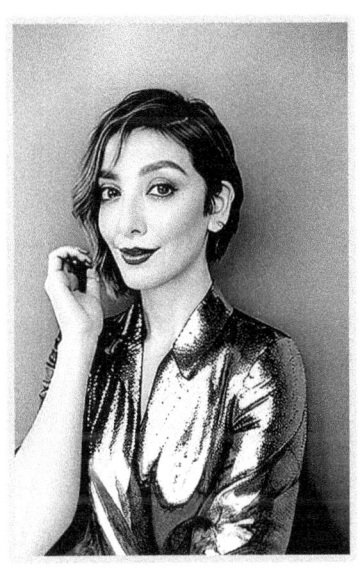

A**IDA I. ASKRY** is a philosopher who delicately intertwines philosophical insights with practical wisdom to explore the depths of human potential, peak performance, and the complexities of human experience.

With a Doctorate in Philosophy focusing on the mind-body connection and a specialization in Leadership and Organizational Development from Harvard Business School, Aida brings a unique and innovative perspective to personal development and systemic change.

Aida is celebrated for her creative and engaging interpretation of complex systems, providing pragmatic insights for those pursuing deep understanding in personal and professional spheres. Her distinctive style combines a playful approach to serious topics, making the exploration of developmental sciences and philosophy an enlightening and enjoyable journey.

Other Titles by the Author

Holistech: A Philosopher's Playbook on the Hidden Art of Flourishing

Published 2023

In her compelling new release, "Holistech," Aida artfully combines elements of her own life story with her philosophical insights, creating a work that is part biography, part guide to living fully. This book draws readers into an engaging journey through the realms of philosophy, biohacking, and peak performance, offering both deep insights and actionable strategies for a richer, more fulfilled life. If you were intrigued by the synthesis of timeless wisdom in "Insight Job," then "Holistech" will provide another illuminating expedition into the art of flourishing.